Carb cycling for weight loss for women

LUCY J. BELL

Table of contents

INTRODUCTION

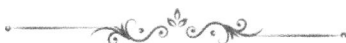

Whenever someone mentions the word "diet" in today's society the first thing that comes to mind is starting to eat less, exercise till exhaustion and probably starve ourselves. The modern concept of female beauty is based on something created artificially in order to promote beauty products and impossible diets. It has all a terrible impact not only on our confidence and self-image, but also on our diets. We decide to chase perfect beauty standards, often at the expense of our health.

What if we could lose weight and have a healthy and pleasant diet? It's possible and this book is the perfect place to start.

The first food that people avoid or remove from their diet when they want to lose weight are the carbs. How often have you decided that bread and pasta were evil products and that were banished from your house? You may have even heard Hollywood stars promote no carbs diets, such as Gwyneth Paltrow, that has made the fight against carbs her brand. But that is absolutely not necessary. You can lose weight AND eat carbs; they are actually necessary for a healthy diet.

Carb cycling is nothing new, it's been used for decades by personal trainers and in the bodybuilding and fitness world. It's a program that can be adapted to every person's needs. It can allow people to not give up their favourite meals. This can help with the mood and the will to continue to eat healthy. How many diets end soon just because people don't see immediate results and have to give up to every tasty food? The utilization of carb cycling as a nutritional approach can fortify one's resolve during the regimen.

In essence, carb cycling can prove to be a potent means of transforming body composition and augmenting physical performance. Nevertheless, it is imperative to consult with a medical expert and integrate carb cycling within a comprehensive, wholesome diet for optimal results. In any case, carb cycling is not a magic formula, it can't make you lose a grand amount of weight in one day. Like for any other diet, perseverance, patience, and willpower are the key. You have to commit yourself fully in order to see results.

This book aims to show you the basics of carbs cycling without confusing you with big terms and incomprehensible recipes. You can see quick results, but you have to ready do the hard work and show up. This book is made to help you reach your goal and guide you through the process with a meal and exercise plan and with plenty of recipes to take inspiration from.

In this book, we will explore the science behind carb cycling, provide meal plans, recipes and workout plans, and discuss tips and strategies for successful implementation. We will also cover frequently asked questions and troubleshooting tips to help you navigate the carb cycling journey. Whether you're a beginner or an experienced pro, this guide will provide the information and resources you need to make carb cycling a successful part of your overall health and fitness plan. It's important to remember, though, that carb cycling is not a one-size-fits-all approach and should be tailored to the individual's goals, activity level, and dietary preferences. Prior to embarking on a carb cycling regimen, it is of utmost importance to solicit the advice of a healthcare professional or a licensed dietician.

This volume, besides rendering an exhaustive analysis of carb cycling, shall also delve into the various advantages that accrue from its implementation, including weight reduction, heightened insulin responsiveness, and augmented energy levels. It should also discuss the different types of carb cycling methods, such as targeted carb cycling and cyclical carb cycling, and explain the science behind how carb cycling works in the body. Lastly, it should address the importance of proper nutrition and exercise in conjunction with carb cycling for optimal results.

PART ONE

CARB CYCLING

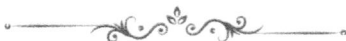

Carbs are famous to be a food to avoid in order to lose weight. They are rumoured to be bad for one's health and people suggest to eliminate them from the diet in order to have a healthy life. But that's not true at all. Carbs are essential for the diet and removing them put the organism under a great amount of stress, putting our health in danger. Low carb diets are dangerous and could increase the possibility to develop cancer, heart problems and kidneys infections. Moreover, it's true that removing carbs allows to lose a lot of weight in a small amount of time, but it's also true that it's possible to regain all if not more weight once you replenish carbs in your diet. Furthermore carbs, especially if taken in the evening could stimulate the production of serotonin, that can help with the relaxation, facilitating sleep.

It is imperative to recognize that carb cycling is not a universal panacea, and may not be suitable for every individual. Those who exhibit sensitivity towards carbohydrates or have a past marked by aberrant eating habits, ought to seek the counsel of a healthcare professional before initiating a carb cycling regimen.

Additionally, carb cycling should be combined with an overall healthy diet that includes a balance of protein, carbohydrates, and healthy fats. Sufficient protein intake is of particular import for those who aim to enhance muscle mass and optimize athletic performance.

Carb cycling is just a diet that allows you to eat healthy, alternating carbs weekly. It's not an eliminatory diet, where carbs are not allowed and banished. Carb cycling is also not a low-fat diet, in fact, the intake of fats is increased on the low carb days, in order to reach the necessary caloric intake level. The key to this program is that the levels of carbs fluctuate during the week, allowing the metabolisms to have a boost and take the necessary amount of energy from the right place.

Carbohydrates are not the maligned sustenance that is commonly perceived, they can prove to be just as instrumental in weight reduction as protein and fats. Every nutrient is necessary to a healthy diet, even carbs. With carb cycling it's even easier to reach your weight goal, let's see how to benefit from this technique and how to lose weight with carb cycling.

1.1. Types of carb cycling

Carb cycling represents a pliant and adaptable nutritional strategy that entails purposeful modulation of carbohydrate consumption to attain specific objectives. There are several different types of carb cycling methods, each with its own set of advantages and disadvantages.

One popular method is targeted carb cycling. This approach involves consuming higher amounts of carbohydrates on days when you are engaging in intense physical activity or training, and lower amounts of carbohydrates on rest days. This is done in order to provide your body with the fuel it needs to perform at its best during workouts, while also allowing for fat loss and muscle growth on rest days.

Another carb cycling method is cyclical carb cycling. This approach involves cycling through periods of high carbohydrate intake and low carbohydrate intake. This can be accomplished through a cyclical alternation between periods of elevated carbohydrate intake and periods of reduced carbohydrate intake, or through a structured regimen of elevated carbohydrate consumption on selected days of the week and diminished carbohydrate consumption on other days. This method is often used by bodybuilders and athletes to help support muscle growth and recovery.

Ultimately, the type of carb cycling method you choose will depend on your individual goals, preferences, and lifestyle.

This book will focus almost exclusively on the target carb cycling, as we think it's the best combination of diet and exercise that is easy to plan for everyone, even for people that have new to diet and workouts plans.

1.2. Understanding macros and macronutrients

When it comes to nutrition and dieting, the terms "macros" and "macronutrients" are often thrown around. But what do they mean and why are they important for carb cycling?

Macros, short for macronutrients, refer to the three main types of nutrients our bodies need in large amounts. Each of these macronutrients plays a specific role in our bodies and are necessary for proper bodily function.

Carbohydrates, being the principal source of energy for the organism, are abundant in numerous edibles, encompassing fruits, vegetables, grains, and sugars. These are the predominant macronutrient that is the focus of attenuation during low-carb days in a carb cycling regimen. The metabolic breakdown of carbohydrates yields glucose, which the body employs as fuel. During periods of high carbohydrate intake, the organism is supplied with a profusion of glucose, which is sequestered in the muscles and liver in the form of glycogen. This glycogen is then used for energy during low-carb days.

Proteins are essential for the growth and repair of our muscles, skin, and other tissues. Proteins, consisting of amino acids that serve as the foundational elements of the organism's tissues, can be procured from a wide range of edibles such as meat, fish, eggs, and dairy products. Adequate protein intake is important for maintaining muscle mass while carb cycling.

Fats are important for hormone production and energy storage. Fats, an essential component of a balanced diet, can be obtained from a diversity of aliments including avocado, nuts, oils, and fatty fish. Additionally, fats play a crucial role in the uptake of fat-soluble vitamins, including vitamin A, D, E, and K. Fats are also an important source of energy during low-carb days.

When adhering to a carb cycling diet, it is essential to attain a harmonious balance of all three macronutrients for optimal fuelling of the body and promotion of weight loss. During periods of elevated carbohydrate intake, emphasis should be placed on obtaining a moderate amount of carbohydrates while concurrently obtaining sufficient amounts of protein and healthy fats.

Conversely, during periods of reduced carbohydrate intake, the focus should be on augmenting protein and healthy fat intake while limiting carbohydrate consumption. It is critical to comprehend the distinct functions of each macronutrient and how they interplay within the body. Carbohydrates supply energy, proteins promote growth and repair, and fats serve as insulation and store energy. By understanding how each macronutrient works in the body, it is easier to make informed decisions about what to eat while carb cycling.

It is also important to track your macronutrient intake while carb cycling. This objective can be achieved by utilizing a food journal or a macronutrient tracking application. Monitoring and documenting macronutrient intake helps to ensure consistency and enables adaptability as circumstances dictate.

In summary, understanding macros and macronutrients is essential for successful carb cycling. By understanding the role of each macronutrient in the body, it is easier to make informed decisions about what to eat. It is also important to track your macronutrient intake to stay on track and make adjustments as needed.

1.3. What are carbs?

Carbohydrates, commonly referred to as saccharides, serve as the primary source of energy for the human body. These macronutrients can be found in a range of plant-based foods, such as bread, pasta, and cereals, as well as dairy products in the form of lactose. Not only do carbohydrates provide energy, but they also impact various biological processes, including immune system function, reproduction, blood clotting, and disease development.

The human body converts carbohydrates into glucose, which functions as the principal energy source for the brain and muscles. Along with proteins and fats, carbohydrates are essential macronutrients that the body requires in substantial quantities.

The recommended daily carbohydrate intake for individuals varies based on several factors, including physical activity levels, body size, and blood sugar control. On average, it is advised that individuals consume a proportion of 45-65% of their total caloric intake in the form of carbohydrates.

According to the Food and Drug Administration (FDA), a 2,000-calorie diet should consist of a daily intake of approximately 275 grams of carbohydrates.

Carbohydrates in food can take several different forms, including dietary fibre, total sugars, and sugar alcohols. Dietary fibre, found in foods such as fruits, vegetables, nuts, seeds, beans, and whole grains, is a type of carbohydrate that the body has difficulty digesting. Total sugars, on the other hand, include naturally occurring sugars in foods such as dairy and added sugars commonly found in baked goods, sweets, and desserts. Sugar alcohols, which are used as reduced-calorie sweeteners in products such as chewing gum, baked goods, and sweets, are a type of carbohydrate that is not fully absorbed by the body and have a sweet taste with fewer calories compared to sugar.

Carbohydrates are a macronutrient that can be classified into two broad categories, simple and complex. Simple carbohydrates, such as monosaccharides and disaccharides, are made up of one or two sugar molecules and provide a quick burst of energy. On the other hand, complex carbohydrates, such as polysaccharides, consist of chains of many sugar molecules and offer sustained energy and a greater array of vitamins, minerals, and fibre.

Examples of simple carbohydrates include white bread, candy, and sugar, while examples of complex carbohydrates include whole grains, fruits, vegetables, and beans. Despite being often demonized, carbohydrates, particularly those derived from natural sources, have numerous health benefits, and can reduce the risk of obesity, heart disease, and type 2 diabetes.

1.4. Definition of carb cycling

The utilization of carb cycling entails fluctuating carbohydrate consumption through alternating periods of high and low ingestion, with the objective of optimally modifying physique composition and enhancing physical performance. As previously established, carbohydrates serve as a vital energy source for all individuals. Carb cycling consist of creating a dietary plan according to each different person, where you may have days of low carbs, but high fat, or days of high fat and low carbs. The alternation of carbs can change daily, weekly, or even monthly. Carb cycling is perfect to suit the needs of the person doing it, but it requires a bit more planning than the other classical diets.[1] The utilization of carb cycling involves alternating the intake of carbohydrates based on the designated day, with the aim of

---

[1] Kubala J., Zambon V., *How carb cycling works and how to do it*, in <<Medical news today>>, 30/03/2021.

optimizing physical appearance and athletic performance. This dietary strategy is often synchronized with physical exertion, necessitating increased consumption of carbohydrates on days that demand greater energy output. By embracing carb cycling, one can enjoy the benefits of a low-carbohydrate diet, without completely forgoing beloved foods.

The fundamental principle behind carb cycling is that, by cyclically consuming a higher quantity of carbohydrates, glycogen stores in both muscles and liver can be replenished, thereby enhancing athletic performance. Moreover, the periodic consumption of increased levels of carbohydrates may augment metabolism, leading to heightened fat oxidation.

Conversely, by intermittently reducing carbohydrate intake, one can mitigate insulin levels and heighten fat oxidation, resulting in a more favourable physique.

It's all about strategy, rather than privation. It's all about changing mentality and understanding finally that carbs are necessary in order to lose weight. Eating carbs will allow you to feel satisfied when you eat and will boost your metabolism, allowing you to have more energy during your workouts. It's a win-win situation.[2]

It's possible to plan the consumption of carbs based on different factors:

- **Training or rest days**→ More carbs during the training days in order to have more energy and low carbs on rest days.

- **Planned reefed**→ Alternate days with high carb meals with days without carbs. The reefed is a strategy that consist of strategically planning, in a long term period, days in which carb assumption is increased.

- **Competition days** → Athletes often increase carbs on days in

---

[2] Pritzker S., Carb Cycling for weight Loss: 21 day meal and exercise plan, Rockridge Press, California, 2021, p. 2.

which are planned matches or competitions.

- Fat levels → The less fat levels the more carbs are increased in the diet.

- Fatisfaction → Psychological satisfaction is fundamental for the success of the diet. To plan high carb days will allow the person to look forward to those days and to "breath again" and "recharge" during a long-term diet.[3]

1.5. The benefits of cycling carbs

Cycling carbs is not only good for fat loss, but also actually very healthy. It can help you regulate your energy intake, control your hunger, and even improve your mental focus and hormonal profile. Let's see how carbs impact the body, so you'll fully understand the benefits of cycling.

We've already seen how stabilizing the blood sugar through the regularization of insulin will help you lose fat, but it will also help you improve your moods and reduce your cravings. All of this is possible by reducing the carbs intake. This cyclical pattern will engender a virtuous cycle, whereby alternating carbohydrate intake leads to increased feelings of well-being and satisfaction, which in turn stimulates continued adherence to healthy dietary habits. It's a win-win situation. Just remember to eat the "good" carbs! Let's see all the benefits closely.

1) Fat burning. When embarking upon a restrictive dietary regimen, an individual may experience a rapid decline in weight in the short-term. However, as time progresses, the rate of weight loss may begin to plateau. This occurs as the hormones within the body, specifically those that regulate appetite and energy expenditure, work to minimize further weight loss. During this phase, the hormone leptin

---

[3] Grimaldi M., *Cos'è il carb cycling e come funziona?,* in <<alimentazione, benessere, attività fisica, salute>>, 4/07/2018, my translation.

comes into play. Leptin, which regulates appetite and energy expenditure, signals the brain that the body is not receiving an adequate caloric intake when its levels are low, leading to a series of physiological changes, such as increased food consumption and decreased calorie burning, a phenomenon known as adaptive thermogenesis. The principles of carb cycling posit that consuming carbohydrates regularly can prevent the body from adapting to this new metabolic state and temporarily increase leptin levels on days with a larger carbohydrate intake, thereby potentially enhancing metabolism and the body's long-term fat-burning capabilities.[4]

2) Improve moods and energy. When starting a diet is easy to lose focus and start the old unhealthy habits, especially if the results are slow. Steady blood sugars will help you with cranky moods and with finding motivation again. Steady blood sugars will make you feel energetic during the day and will make you feel happier even if you're doing a diet. When you eliminate carbs from your diet is natural to feel tired, sad, and unsatisfied. Carb cycling will allow you to avoid the brain fog and fatigue of a restrictive diet, providing you energy for the body. Through the glucose you'll be sustained for every moment of your day. Remember to avoid processed carbs, in order to avoid crashes. If you choose high-fibre, whole food carb sources and spread them out throughout the day, you'll feel full longer, energized during the day and feel alert and focused.

It is imperative to note that abruptly lowering carbohydrate consumption, particularly for those habituated to consuming a significant amount of carbohydrates on a daily basis, may result in feelings of fatigue and nervousness. But it's momentary, it's a sign that your body is getting used to the right amount of carbs and of sugar in your blood, so don't give up and trust the process![5]

---

[4] Younkin L., *Carb Cycling diet – what is it? Does It work?*, in <<EatingWell>>, 12/11/2022.
[5] Dustin M., The Everything Guide to the Carb Cycling Diet: An effective Diet plan to lose weight and boost your metabolism, Simon and Schuster, U.S.A., 2016.

3) Hormones and muscles. Reducing and managing the carbs intake can also be positive on your hormonal profile. Believe it or not, it can be very positive for your sex hormone production, especially if you start losing fat.

The human body stores glycogen in the muscles and liver as a readily available source of energy. During periods of low-carbohydrate intake in the context of carb cycling, glycogen storage becomes limited. To mitigate this, high-carbohydrate days are incorporated to replenish glycogen stores within the muscles. This, in turn, may enhance physical performance and mitigate the breakdown of muscle tissue.

4) Cycling carbs has also a last benefit: you can still enjoy your favourite foods (although in moderation). On special occasions, birthdays, or celebrations you can make fit into your plan every kind of meal. On high carb days you can eat pasta or pizza as a treat and you'll still see the results. Just remember the calorie intake. The important is to eat the right number of calories. We've said that you should eat "good" carbs, however, that does not indicate an inability to relish a festive gathering or a noteworthy occasion.. It's ok to eat processed carbs once in a while, the important thing is doing it on high carb days and to respect the calories intake of the day. With some self-control is possible to enjoy any birthday or event with carb cycling.

Life is meant to be enjoyed and this type of diet can help you find the perfect balance.

1.6. Cons of carb cycling

Carb cycling might also have some cons if you don't plan ahead and don't focus on the program.

1) Exaggerate with carbs. Adhering to a cyclical carbohydrate regimen is challenging, owing to the problematic nature of determining the appropriate amount of carbohydrates to consume during both high and low carbohydrate phases. It can also take a lot of your time to track carbs and other macronutrients.

2) Peril of developing an unhealthy relationship with food. Maintaining this kind of diet long term can be really tricky. You might develop huge cravings during low carb days and binge eat on high carb days. Also, this diet doesn't take into consideration the appetite of a person. Not everyone is starving after a workout and might be hungrier on the most boring days.

1.7. How to stay focused on the program

The first thing that comes to mind when starting a diet is "I'm going to be hungry all the time". That's a common belief, but it's not true at all. During carb cycling you'll consume the right number of calories that you'll need during the day. But hunger is a tricky thing. there are two types of hunger that you need to recognize: physical hunger and emotional hunger. Physical hunger is about your body telling you its needs and is a healthy type of hunger. Emotional hunger is very common and hard to recognize. You usually feel emotional hunger when you're stressed, sad, bored or even happy. Emotional hunger is the worst enemy for anyone that starts a diet, you'll be tempted to eat food that you don't need and that is not healthy. Knowing you're on a diet can actually be even more triggering.

Therefore, it is crucial to acquire the ability to differentiate between emotional starvation prior to embarking on the cyclical carbohydrate regimen. You can try to go a long time without eating one day, it will be hard, and I suggest to do it on a very busy day, so you'll have less time to think about food. You'll learn self-control and how to recognize the signs of physical hunger. Stress factors and a chaotic life can increase emotional hunger. Try to reduce stress, to regulate sleep and drink plenty of water. If you feel hungry try to stop for a moment and ask yourself "Am I really hungry? Is it coming from my body? Or am I just bored/upset/stressed?". These tips can help you with the craving and, hopefully, after the first day (the hardest ones) the effects of carb cycling will kick in and you'll feel less hungry and more satisfied.[6]

1.8. The functioning of carb cycling

Low carbs diets have their pros and are usually very effective in fat loss. However, they are advocated for a circumscribed duration. Doing a low carb diet for too long will leave you without carbs to burn during your workout session. This will increase the danger of injury and will compromise the immune system. Low carb diets will also increase the possibility to regain all the lost weight rapidly once you start eating carbs again. High carbs diets are perfect to maintain a right amount of energy in your body, allowing you to give your best during the workout sessions. With carb cycling you'll lose weight without risking your health.

Carb cycling endeavours to assist individuals in attaining their weight and physical fitness objectives through oscillating between periods of low and high carbohydrate consumption. On days where carbohydrate intake is minimal, the organism relies on the utilization of already present glycogenic carbohydrates within the body.

Decreasing the quantity of carbohydrates ingested leads to a reduction in insulin secretion, thereby augmenting the body's sensitivity to the insulin present in circulation. As a result, on high carbohydrate intake days, the body primarily utilizes carbohydrates as a source of energy rather than facilitating their storage as adipose tissue. High carbs days booster your metabolism, allowing you to have more energy. They allow you to recharge your organism. Enhancing one's metabolism through this method will also result in the generation of leptin, a hormone which will instruct the central nervous system to expend more energy. It is imperative that high carbohydrate intake days be synchronized with days of exercise, while low carbohydrate

---

[6] Ibidem.

intake days are scheduled on rest days where a diminished energy demand is present. Using the carbs you eat is an essential part the carb cycling program and it's also the reason why it works.[7]

But let's see examine more in depth this process. First of all, everyone that suggest a low carb diet points fingers at insulin as one of the worst hormones, claiming that it's programmed to make us fat. The truth is that insulin doesn't make us fat, but let's see why and how carb cycling can use this hormone to make us lose weight.

We've already seen what carbs are, let's see what happens to them once they are consumed. The whole process begins with the digestion. The carbs are divided into single molecules of glucose. Glucose serves as an energy source for the organism. The rate of glucose utilization can vary and is contingent upon the category of carbohydrate in question. Simple carbs will be digested more quickly than complex carbs, as they can be broken down faster. Glucose will be absorbed in the bloodstream after the digestion and will be stored in adipose tissue (fat cells) or will be carried to places that need energy. Eating a lot of carbs will elevate the sugar levels in the blood. This will activate the response of the body, that will signal the blood sugar increase to the pancreas, that will release insulin in order to help clear the blood of glucose and help get it stored properly.[8]

Initially, those who advocate for a low carbohydrate diet often characterize insulin as an unfavourable hormone, alleging that it is designed to cause obesity. The reality, however, is that insulin does not induce obesity, but we shall examine how and why carb cycling can harness this hormone to facilitate weight loss. Insulin is a hormone that transports nutrients to cells via the bloodstream. Upon consuming food, it is divided into various substances that insulin, secreted by the pancreas, conveys into the bloodstream. As the nutrients permeate the

---

[7] Pritzker S., Carb Cycling for weight Loss: 21 day meal and exercise plan, Rockridge Press, California, 2021, p. 3.
[8] Dustin M., The Everything Guide to the Carb Cycling Diet: An effective Diet plan to lose weight and boost your metabolism, Simon and Schuster, U.S.A., 2016.

cells, insulin secretion gradually declines until absorption is complete, after which insulin remains at a low baseline level.

This metabolic cycle takes place every time food is consumed, causing insulin levels to continuously fluctuate throughout the day.

Insulin is essential for the proper functioning of the body, but unfortunately, it also impedes the degradation of adipocytes and encourages the formation of body fat. This occurs as insulin instructs the body to temporarily cease fat metabolism and instead utilize the energy from the recently consumed food. Additionally, insulin facilitates the storage of a portion of the available energy as body fat. Although, when you consistently eat too many carbs and the sugar levels in your blood are constantly high, the body requires always more insulin to handle the too much sugar, this can cause your body to lose the sensitivity to insulin, pushing the pancreas to produce always more insulin. You'll then need more and more insulin to do the same amount of work less insulin would have done. Eventually tour pancreas would not be able to produce enough insulin.[9]

So, we have the impression that the more we eat, the more the insulin levels rise and the more we store fat and get fatter. And we are told that the less we eat, the less the insulin levels rise and the more we lose weight. It sounds logical, but the problem is the energy disbalance that this can cause.

Energy balance refers to the correlation between the amount of energy ingested and the amount expended.

This interdependence determines the alteration in weight over time and holds primacy over any considerations related to insulin or other hormones. To put it simply, substantial accumulation of fat is not feasible without a consistent surplus of energy for storage as fat.

Conversely, significant fat loss cannot occur without maintaining the body in a substantial energy deficit, thus compelling it to draw from

---

[9] Ibidem.

its adipose reserves to sustain its metabolic functions. This concept is validated by studies that indicate that, so long as protein intake is equalized, fat loss occurs similarly with both high carbohydrate and low carbohydrate diets.

Carb cycling can help improve your insulin sensitivity. With the long periods of low carbs intake, you can allow your body to reset itself and learn to use insulin properly again.

Individuals may also decrease their susceptibility to insulin resistance by incorporating nutritious carbohydrates into their diet, preserving appropriate sleep patterns, and engaging in consistent physical activity.

Nutritious carbohydrates encompass fruit, vegetables, leguminous plants, whole grains, and selected grain-based products. These foodstuffs comprise essential vitamins, minerals, fibre, and crucial phytochemicals.

So, carb cycling helps you lose weight not really thanks to the use of carbs, the key to fat loss is the protein intake and the energy balance that are the result of said alternation of carbs.

PART TWO

CARB CYCLING APPLIED

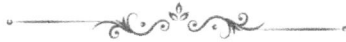

Carb cycling requires a bit more of planning and can be overwhelming at first. Don't give up and follow the advice of this book. It'll be much easier once you start.

A widely utilized technique of carb cycling entails alternating between days of elevated carbohydrate intake and days of diminished carbohydrate consumption. On days of elevated carbohydrate intake, a higher quantity of carbohydrates, typically in the range of 2-3 grams per pound of body weight, are consumed. On low carb days, you would consume a lower amount of carbohydrates, usually around 0.5-1 gram per pound of body weight.

Another popular method of carb cycling is to alternate between high carb days, moderate carb days, and low carb days. On high carb days, you would consume a higher amount of carbohydrates, usually around 2-3 grams per pound of body weight. On moderate carb days, you would consume a moderate amount of carbohydrates, usually around 1-2 grams per pound of body weight. On low carb days, you would consume a lower amount of carbohydrates, usually around 0.5-1 gram per pound of body weight.

A classic carb cycling week program can be divided into:

- Two high carbs days;

- Two days in which carbs are reduced a bit;

- Three low carbs days.

The consumption of proteins can be the same for all of the seven days, but the fat consumption has to vary, depending on the carbs consumption. On high carbs days the consumption of fat is drastically reduced, on the contrary, on low carbs days the consumption of fat must increase.

In any case, the plan can change according to the goals of each person. If your goals is to lose weight fast you could switch to 5 low carb days alternated to just 2 high carb days. For individuals seeking to augment muscle mass and who are professional athletes, a variation of the carb cycling approach could involve switching to five days of elevated carbohydrate intake, alternating with only two days of reduced carbohydrate consumption. It's important though to alternate the days correctly an not have too many high carb days all together. You can also decide to start with a plan and adjust it throughout the program in order to archive the best results.

2.1. High carb days

High carb days must coincide with your workout days, this is to help you have the maximum energy when needed. For those who do not have a workout regimen, scheduling high carbohydrate intake days can be determined based on individual preference, with care taken to avoid excessive consecutive days of elevated carbohydrate consumption. You can plan them on the weekend or base them according to social events or birthdays.

High carb days can also help with the cravings and will prevent you from giving up before seeing the results. On higher carb days the major intake of carbs can come from rice, pasta, fruit, and potatoes. The protein intake should be the same of low carb days and fat source should be lowered since the higher carb intake will increase the total calories.

Let's calculate the macros for a high carb day:

<u>Carbs</u>: your weight x 1.5 grams= grams of carbs

<u>Protein intake</u>: The number of grams of protein can be calculated by multiplying your body weight by 0.6.

<u>Fat intake</u>: The number of grams of fats can be calculated by multiplying your body weight by 0.25.

It is imperative to recall that carbohydrates and proteins both possess four calories per gram, while fats boast nine calories per gram.

Consequently, it is crucial to calculate the macro-nutrient distribution in terms of calories:

<u>Carbs</u>: your macros x 4= calories from carbs

<u>Proteins</u>: your macros x 4= calories from protein

<u>Fat</u>: your macros x 9= calories from fat[10]

Now let's make an example, believe me, even if it's math, it's really simple.

Susanna weighs 154 pounds:

<u>Carbs</u>: 154 x 1.5 grams= 231 grams x 4= 924 calories

<u>Protein</u>: 154 x 0.6 grams= 92.4 grams x 4= 369.6 calories

<u>Fat</u>: 154 x 0.25= 38.5 grams x 9= 346.5 calories

The total daily caloric intake for Susanna on a high carbohydrate day should be 1,640 calories.

2.2. Low carb days

These high carbohydrate days facilitate the utilization of adipose tissue as a source of energy and enhance insulin sensitivity, both of which are crucial factors in the reduction of body fat. Meanwhile, low

---

[10] Pritzker S., Carb Cycling for weight Loss: 21 day meal and exercise plan, Rockridge Press, California, 2021, p. 3.

carbohydrate days are ideal for low-intensity physical activity, such as a leisurely stroll, as the energy demands during such activities are minimal. On these days the carbs intake should be set very low. One thing to remember is to avoid drinking anything with an excessive amount of carbs, as this can defeat the purpose of a low carb day. On these days it's important to increase the intake of fat, in order to maintain an equilibrium in the calorie's intake.

Let's calculate the macros for a low carb day:

Carbs: your weight x 0.5 grams= grams of carbs

Protein intake: Multiply your mass by 0.6 to determine the quantity of protein in grams.

Fat: your weight x 0.4= grams of fat

Let's calculate your macros in calories:

Carbs: your macros x 4= calories from carbs

Proteins: your macros x 4= calories from protein

Fat: your macros x 9= calories from fat[11]

And now, just like we've done for high carb days, let's make an example.

Susanna weighs, just like before, 154 pounds:

Carbs: 154 x 0.5 grams= 77 grams x 4= 308 calories

Protein: 154 x 0.6 grams= 92.4 grams x 4= 369.6 calories

Fat: 154 x 0.4= 61.6 grams x 9= 554.4 calories

Susanna's total daily calorie intake for a low carb day should be: 1,232 calories.

It must be emphasized that no calculation or approximation will ever be entirely precise, as each individual is unique and has distinct metabolic rates, lifestyles, and habits. These variables must be taken

---

[11] Ibidem.

into consideration when making such estimations. However, you can consider this a starting point and then adjust the plan and the numbers later.

2.3. What to eat

Carb cycling prioritizes the modulation of macronutrient (carbohydrates, proteins, and fats) intake, rather than a restrictive regimen on specific foods, thereby affording room for a diverse array of dietary options. However, for maximum fat reduction and to thwart the prospect of weight regain, it is crucial to heed the quality of the foodstuffs consumed. High carb days should not be misinterpreted as a license to consume any and all comestibles, including junk food. It's important to choose the right carbs. It's also important to remember that for an effective fat loss is essential a calorie deficit. If you simply substitute the carbs with more proteins or fats on your low carb days, you will still gain more weight instead of losing it. Carb cycling will help you lose weight only if you stick to the right calories and to the right amount of exercise. When one consistently consumes an energy surplus, they shall experience an increase in body weight as the intake of calories surpasses the body's ability to utilize them. For fat loss, a calorie deficit is a must. Let's explain this with the first law of thermodynamics: energy cannot be created or destroyed, only transformed. If you take more calories than your body can consume, you'll gain body fat. If you consume more calories than the ones you take, your body will have to take energy somewhere else, and it will take it from the stored fat.

So, you don't have to eliminate a product from your diet, but you have to control the quantities. Carb cycling can also help boost the metabolism and help you take energy from the right place. During high carb days you have to remember that quality is equally important to quantity in this diet. It is imperative to be discerning in selecting the variety of carbohydrates one ingests. If the carbs you eat on high carb days are highly processed, you might suffer blood sugar crashes that come from a high dose of processed carbs. These crashes tend to leave you feeling tired and hungry. If you eat sweets or candy, you'll know that they'll make you feel full and satisfied just for a few moments, then you'll be tired and even more hungry. On high carb days is important to take the carbs intake from "good", non-processed carbs.

The best "good" carbs are:

Whole grains: those are really healthy and are beneficial for the health. A few examples are: whole rice, oat, quinoa.

Tubers: potatoes and sweet potatoes.

Unprocessed fruits: fruit is made of sugar, is healthy sugar, but if you're worried about blood sugar crashes you have to pay attention to the quantity of fruit you decide to eat during the day.

Legumes.

Examining the "bad" carbohydrates that one ought to evade. Adverse saccharides are expeditiously metabolized saccharides that engender a prompt elevation of the blood glucose levels.

White sugar, bread, pasta, and flour: eat whole grain pasta or bread, whole wheat couscous, or quinoa rather than white pasta, bread and flour.

Sugary drinks and juices: replace fizzy drinks or fruit juices made from concentrate with water or natural fruit juices.

Cakes, candy, and cookies: choose whole fruits instead of foods that are high in added sugar, such as cakes or cookies.

Other processed foods: you can try eating healthy snacks like dried fruit.

Let's see an example of menu for each day.

High carb day:

Breakfast: 2 eggs + 70 gr. rye bread + 150 gr. fruit

Lunch: 200 gr. of sweet potatoes + 200 gr. of fish + raw fennel

Snack: 150 gr. of fruit with coconut flakes and mixed seeds

Dinner: 70 gr. of whole rice + 150 gr. of curry chicken + 200 gr. of vegetables

Low carb day:

Breakfast: 2 eggs + 2 slices of ham + mixed berries

Lunch: 200 gr. of salmon + salad

Snack: 30 gr. of dark chocolate + 20 gr. of walnuts

Dinner: mixed salad + 150 gr. of turkey + a half of avocado

2.4. Food shopping and preparation

Grocery shopping is really important if you decide to start with carb cycling. Planning ahead is fundamental and having the right ingredients at home is the starting point of the whole program. If you don't plan ahead you might find yourself in difficult situations. If you return home after a hard day of work and don't find the right products in your fridge you might be tempted to eat unhealthy food or even order takeout. Your willpower will be tested, so it's better to plan the weekly meals ahead, in order to have all the things that you need. When creating your meal plan think about easy and enjoyable recipes. At the end of the book you'll find some easy recipe you can take inspiration from. You can plan your meals, go grocery shopping and preparing all at once. You can then store the meals and reheat them when it's time to eat. Of course, if you have a flexible schedule and you like to cook, you can try new and more complex recipes.

When one adheres to a strategy of anticipatory preparation, such as cooking and pre-assembling all provisions, it becomes significantly more effortless to abide by the regimen, necessitating only an exertion of discipline and mastery over one's inclinations.

2.5. Easy carbs substitutions

As we've said in this book carbohydrates are an essential macronutrient that provide our bodies with energy and fuel for physical activity. However, consuming too many carbohydrates can lead to weight gain and other health issues. While high-carb days are important for replenishing glycogen stores and providing energy, it's important to choose the right types of carbohydrates. Whole grains, fruits, vegetables, and legumes are better options than processed foods, white flour, and added sugars.

By incorporating more whole foods and natural sweeteners, you can increase your intake of vitamins, minerals, and fibre, while also reducing your intake of added sugars and preservatives.

Another important factor to consider is portion control. Even healthy carbohydrates can add up quickly if you eat too much. Be mindful of serving sizes and pay attention to how you feel after eating. If you find yourself feeling overly full or sluggish, it may be a sign that you have exceeded your carb needs for the day.

Remember that the key to successful carb cycling is finding a balance that works for you. By experimenting with different carb substitutions and paying attention to how your body responds, you can find the perfect balance of carbohydrates to fuel your body and support your goals. It may take some trial and error, but with patience and perseverance, you'll be able to find a carb cycling plan that works for you.

The substitution options listed above are a great starting point for incorporating healthier carb choices into your high-carb days.

- Instead of white rice, try quinoa or cauliflower rice for a lower-carb option.

- Instead of regular pasta, try whole wheat pasta or vegetable-based pasta such as zucchini noodles (zoodles) or spaghetti squash.

- Instead of white bread, try whole wheat or sprouted grain bread.

- Instead of regular potatoes, try sweet potatoes, yams, or cauliflower mash.

- Instead of sugary snacks and desserts, try fresh fruit or low-sugar alternatives such as dark chocolate, berries, or a small serving of homemade trail mix with nuts, seeds, and dried fruit.

- Instead of regular soda, try sparkling water with a splash of juice or a low-calorie alternative such as diet soda.

- Instead of regular pizza, try cauliflower crust pizza or make a pizza with a whole wheat crust and lots of vegetables.

- Instead of regular ice cream, try low-calorie alternatives such as frozen yogurt or sorbet.

- Instead of processed cereals, try oatmeal, quinoa flakes, or chia seed pudding for a more nutrient-dense option.

- Instead of regular flour, try almond flour, coconut flour, or chickpea flour for a lower-carb option.

- Instead of white sugar, try natural sweeteners such as honey, maple syrup, or stevia.

- Instead of regular crackers, try seed crackers, rice cakes or low-carb crackers.

- Instead of regular milk, try almond milk, soy milk, or coconut milk for a lower-carb option.

- Instead of regular yogurt, try Greek yogurt or coconut yogurt for a lower-carb option.

- Instead of regular beer, try light beer or hard seltzers that are lower in carbs.

- Instead of regular hummus, try cauliflower hummus or avocado hummus for a lower-carb option.

- Instead of regular granola, try homemade granola made with nuts, seeds, and low-sugar sweeteners.

- Instead of regular lasagne, try zucchini lasagne, eggplant lasagne or portobello mushroom lasagne.

- Instead of regular French fries, try sweet potato fries as a high-carb substitution. They have a lower glycaemic index than regular potatoes, which means they'll provide a more sustained source of energy.

- Instead of conventional rice that is low in carbohydrates is cauliflower rice. This provides a means of incorporating more vegetables into one's diet by simply shredding the florets of a cauliflower in a food processor or procuring pre-processed cauliflower rice. This can serve as a foundation for dishes such as sautés, stews, and even as a substitute for rice in preferred culinary creations.

Remember that these are just suggestions and it's important to find what works for you and your dietary needs. Carbohydrates are essential for energy and well-being, but it's important to choose the right types in the right amounts.

During periods of low carbohydrate intake, it may prove challenging to locate substitutes for the high-carbohydrate provisions that one may be habituated to consuming. However, there are many delicious and satisfying low-carb options that you can incorporate into your diet. These include using vegetables as substitutes for traditional high-carb foods, such as using lettuce leaves or Portobello mushrooms as wraps or buns, using spaghetti squash or zucchini noodles as pasta, and using cauliflower rice as a rice substitute These permutations can facilitate adhesion to your saccharide-restrictive regimen while concurrently relishing delectable and satiating nourishment. Additionally, there are other low-carb alternatives that you can use in your cooking, such as almond flour and coconut flour instead of wheat flour in baking recipes, using avocado or Greek yogurt as a replacement for mayonnaise or sour cream in dips and dressings, and using berries or nuts as a sweetener instead of sugar. Furthermore, there are also low-carb protein options such as chicken, fish, eggs, and tofu. These substitutions can help you to create tasty and healthy meals without sacrificing on flavour or satisfaction.

Here's a list that can help you find the perfect substitution, according to your tastes.

Lettuce wraps: Instead of using bread or a tortilla, try using lettuce leaves to wrap your sandwich or burrito fillings. Romaine lettuce and butter lettuce are great options that can provide a satisfying crunch. Lettuce is also a low-carb alternative to taco shells. They're made by using lettuce leaves such as Romaine, butter lettuce or iceberg lettuce as a wrapper for your favourite taco fillings.

Zucchini noodles: Zucchini spirals, colloquially referred to as "zoodles", serve as a salient low-carb substitute for pasta. They can be fashioned via a spiralizing implement or a planer and present a palatable means of incorporating increased amounts of greens into one's nutritional regimen.

Cauliflower pizza crust: A cauliflower crust is a great low-carb alternative to traditional pizza dough. It's made by grating cauliflower and then mixing it with eggs and cheese to form a dough. It's lower in carbs, calories and gluten-free, but still delicious.

Portobello mushroom caps: Portobello mushroom caps can be used as a low-carb alternative to bread or buns. They can be grilled or sautéed and used as a base for burgers, sandwiches, or even as a pizza crust.

Cabbage leaves: Cabbage leaves can be used as a low-carb alternative to wraps, tacos shells, and sandwich bread. They present an optimal selection for individuals seeking to augment their ingestion of horticultural edibles and are additionally of low caloric content.

Spaghetti squash: this option is a saccharide-restrictive substitute for pasta. Upon culinary preparation, the pulpy interior of the gourd dissociates into slender, spaghetti-resembling filaments, rendering it a superior choice for spaghetti dishes or as a pasta surrogate in any culinary formula.

Eggplant lasagne: Eggplant lasagne is a great low-carb alternative to traditional lasagne. It is fabricated through the utilization of slender cross-sectional slices of aubergine as a pasta surrogate, thereby rendering it an advantageous choice for individuals vigilant of their saccharide intake.

Spinach wraps: Spinach wraps are a low-carb alternative to traditional flour or corn tortillas. They're made from spinach, eggs, and cheese, and can be filled with your favourite sandwich or burrito fillings.

Broccoli rice: Broccoli rice is a great low-carb alternative to traditional rice. It's made by grating or pulsing broccoli in a food processor until it resembles rice-like consistency. It can be used as a substitute for rice in dishes such as stir-fry or in salads.

Cucumber boats: Cucumber boats are a low-carb alternative to bread or crackers. They're made by hollowing out cucumber slices and filling them with your favourite dip or spread.

Portobello mushroom burger buns: Portobello mushroom caps can be used as a low-carb alternative to burger buns. They're large, meaty, and can be grilled or sautéed to provide a delicious and healthy alternative to traditional buns.

Cauliflower rice: this is an interesting alternative to traditional rice. It's made by grating or pulsing cauliflower in a food processor until it resembles rice-like consistency. It can be used as a substitute for rice in dishes such as stir-fry, in salads or as a side dish.

Almond flour pancakes: Almond flour pancakes are a low-carb alternative to traditional pancakes. They're made by using almond flour instead of wheat flour and can be flavoured with your favourite sweeteners and spices.

Coconut flour cookies: Coconut flour cookies are a low-carb alternative to traditional wheat flour cookies. They're made by using coconut flour instead of wheat flour and can be flavoured with your favourite sweeteners, spices and nuts.

Avocado toast: Avocado toast is a low-carb alternative to traditional bread toast. It's made by mashing avocado on top of toasted bread, and can be flavoured with your favourite seasonings, herbs, and spices.

2.6. The 7-day plan

As we've said before, carb cycling will require a lot of planning and preparation beforehand. Limiting carbs is not something that we're familiar with and it's really complicated. It cannot be improvised. If you don't start planning the carb cycling and don't write down your weekly if not monthly plan is easier to give up and start eating unhealthy food again.

Never forget that the quality of food is important just like the preparation of the program. Don't eat junk food on the high carb days, it will put at risk all the progress you've made till then.

When starting to program your plan start with no carb days, paired with non-intense activities. Don't do your toughest and most strenuous exercise day on your no carb day, but opposite instead.

Following the no carb days plan some low carb day and just at the end the high carb days. On your high carb days do the most exhausting workouts, so to use and burn the energy that the carbs give you. Physical exercise in these days can involve 30 minutes of lifting weights at the gym, going for long run or hiking. Intense exercise depletes glycogen and primes your body to absorb nutrients. Low intensity activities, such as slow walking, don't have the same effect. Resistance exercise is eminently suitable for saccharide oscillation due to the creation of a milieu where the organism will be predisposed to utilize nutrients for rejuvenation and amelioration, as opposed to their sequestration as adipose tissue. This type of training causes micro-damage to your muscles, so those few hours after a training session are a great time to enjoy your carbs, as your body will use them to recover.

If you exercise a lot and follow a workout plan, it's fundamental that you plan the high carb days in the same days of the workouts because those are the days in which you'll need more energy. When you train you use glucose, so it's a perfect time for carbs intake.[12]

If you train three days a week, then those three days are going to become your high carb days. If you train more than three days a week then you'll have to do some thinking. Reflect on which are the most intensive workouts and plan the high carb days on those days. If you have cardio days or if you train the lower-body then your body is going to ask you for more energy than in the days in which you train the upper body.

Following the period of elevated saccharide intake, revert to the state of saccharide-restrictive intake prior to re-engaging in the state of saccharide deprivation once more. Then, repeat the cycle.

Individuals may opt to occasionally abstain from the regimen to avoid the necessity of saccharide enumeration and to mitigate burnout, however, such decisions are contingent upon the individual's personal discipline and willpower.

So, the first step to take when planning your meals is deciding how many high carb days you will have each week and when to plan them. As we've said, carb cycling is not a strict diet, but a mindset, a theory to apply to your everyday life. Depending on how many workouts you do, you can decide to have a minimum of two high carb days to a maximum of four. If you're new to diets and find difficult to follow them I suggest starting with four high carb days, regardless of how much you exercise. If you've tried many diets and find difficult to lose weight, start with just two high carb days.

---

[12] Dustin M., The Everything Guide to the Carb Cycling Diet: An effective Diet plan to lose weight and boost your metabolism, Simon and Schuster, U.S.A., 2016.

When you plan your meals is important to remember a few things and to avoid some combinations. After workouts it's better to consume carbs and proteins, you will be able to absorb them quickly. If you want to stay full for a while, then the best option is proteins with fats. The combination you have to avoid is carbs with fats. Carbs raise your insulin and if the only nutrients your body can find are glucose and fatty acids, those will go straight to your fat cells. Of course, if that happens, it's now the end of the world, you won't regain instantly all the lost weight and you won't lose your progress, but if you want to optimize your results, you have to pay attention and avoid that combination as much as you can.

There actually four main carb cycling plans that you can choose of get inspiration from, depending on your needs and habits.

1) Easy Cycle

This plan serves as an appropriate starting point for a saccharide oscillation journey. Simply put, this will assist in acclimatization to the schedules of low and elevated saccharide intake and will familiarize one with the edibles permissible for saccharide cycling. The advantage of this cyclical plan lies in the allowance of a singular indulgent repast four days per week. These indulgent repasts can consist of any food item desired, whether it be pizza, frozen confection, pastry, or even cured pork belly, provided they are not consumed during the evening meal. This permits the satisfaction of any gustatory desires, albeit necessitating a delay until the elevated saccharide days. If adherence to the fundamental guidelines of saccharide cycling appears formidable, it is advisable to first attune one's body with this plan.

A sample 7-Day of this plan may appear as follows:

Day 1: Low carb day

Day 2: High carb day, included of one reward meal

Day 3: Low carb day

Day 4: High carb day, included of one reward meal

Day 5: Low carb day

Day 6: High carb day, included of one reward meal

Day 7: High carb day, included of one reward meal

This cyclical approach pertains to the development of dietary habits and the establishment of a saccharide cycling foundation. It is imperative to continuously recall that all nourishment during this cycle ought to be in comparatively modest portions than one's customary consumption. Though substantial reduction in body mass and adipose tissue may not be immediately achieved, weight loss shall ensue and serve as a catalyst for a more remarkable odyssey. For certain individuals whose primary objective is to sustain weight and cultivate a salubrious lifestyle, the ameliorated regimen has been established as one of the most efficacious dietary plans.

2) Classic Cycle

For individuals seeking to achieve rapid and sustained weight loss, the Classic Cycle may be a more favourable option than the Easy Cycle. This iteration of the cyclical dietary approach involves stringent differentiation between low and high carbohydrate days, precluding the inclusion of reward meals. Despite this, the Classic Cycle offers a weekly indulgence day, in which caloric intake can surpass the typical daily limit by up to 1,000 calories. It is imperative, however, to abstain from indulging during the evening repast.

A sample 7-Day of this plan may appear as follows:

Day 1: Low carb day

Day 2: High carb day

Day 3: Low carb day

Day 4: High carb day

Day 5: Low carb day

Day 6: High carb day

Day 7: Reward Day

This Cycle not only augments the speed and consistency of weight loss but also enables greater introspection and awareness of the physiological effects of alternating low and high carbohydrate regimes. As a natural consequence of these dietary changes, some individuals may experience symptoms such as nausea and headaches, though they are typically transitory in nature. Adherence to the Classic Cycle can be sustained throughout the entire weight reduction journey or one may choose to graduate to another cyclical plan.

3) Turbo Cycle

For those seeking a rapid reduction in weight, the Turbo Cycle constitutes the optimal plan. This carb cycling regimen yields the quickest weight loss among the available quartet of cycles, as it expedites metabolic rates with unparalleled alacrity.

A sample 7-Day of this plan may appear as follows:

Day 1: Low carb day

Day 2: Low carb day

Day 3: High carb day

Day 4: Low carb day

Day 5: Low carb day

Day 6: High carb day

Day 7: Reward Day

4) Fit Cycle

For individuals seeking a weight loss regimen that is compatible with demanding physical activities, the Fit Cycle is a desirable 7-day program. With the fundamental concepts of carb cycling, this plan facilitates fat reduction, while concurrently supplying the organism with the requisite sustenance and energy for strenuous endeavours. For athletes who continuously engage in physical exercise or those who undergo rigorous training sessions that endure for extended periods, the Fit Cycle will preserve optimal form and readiness for any eventuality.

A sample 7-Day of this plan may appear as follows:

Day 1: High carb day

Day 2: High carb day

Day 3: Low carb day

Day 4: High carb day

Day 5: High carb day

Day 6: Low carb day

Day 7: Reward Day

The Fit Cycle, though less effective in inducing rapid weight loss as compared to the Turbo Cycle, is particularly suitable for those who strive to sustain their athletic performance. If a decline in athletic capabilities is perceived, supplementing, or incorporating meal replacement shakes into one's regimen may prove advantageous, though it will not necessarily amplify weight loss if that is the objective.

Now that we've seen the most common carb cycling plans, let's remember that a carb cycling plan can be tailored to fit an individual's specific goals and needs. Let's see in the practical an example of a classic weekly carb cycling plan, in order to give you an idea of how to build your weekly menu:

Monday: Low Carb Day

Breakfast: Egg omelette with spinach and feta

Snack: Cottage cheese with berries

Lunch: Grilled chicken with mixed greens and a side of avocado

Snack: Boiled egg with a few almonds

Dinner: Grilled steak with broccoli and a side salad

Tuesday: High Carb Day

Breakfast: Oatmeal with fruit

Snack: Apple with almond butter

Lunch: Brown rice with chicken and vegetables

Snack: Greek yogurt with berries

Dinner: Sweet potato with grilled salmon and mixed greens

Wednesday: Low Carb Day

Breakfast: Egg and cheese breakfast burrito with spinach and avocado

Snack: Cottage cheese with berries

Lunch: Grilled chicken with mixed greens and a side of avocado

Snack: Hard-boiled egg with a handful of almonds

Dinner: Grilled pork tenderloin with cauliflower rice and steamed vegetables

Thursday: High Carb Day

Breakfast: Whole wheat toast with peanut butter and banana

Snack: Apple with almond butter

Lunch: Whole wheat pasta with turkey meatballs and marinara sauce

Snack: Greek yogurt with berries

Dinner: Quinoa with roasted vegetables and grilled chicken

Friday: Low Carb Day

Breakfast: Scrambled eggs with diced vegetables

Snack: Cottage cheese with berries

Lunch: Grilled chicken with mixed greens and a side of avocado

Snack: Hard-boiled egg with a handful of almonds

Dinner: Grilled shrimp with zucchini noodles and a side salad

Saturday: High Carb Day (Reward Day)

Breakfast: Whole wheat pancakes with fresh fruit and turkey bacon

Snack: Apple with almond butter

Lunch: Whole wheat pita with falafel and tzatziki sauce

Snack: Greek yogurt with berries

Dinner: Baked sweet potato with black bean and corn chili

Sunday: High Carb Day

Breakfast: Whole wheat toast with peanut butter and banana

Snack: Apple with almond butter

Lunch: Whole wheat pizza with turkey sausage and vegetables

Snack: Greek yogurt with berries

Dinner: Baked potato with grilled steak and mixed vegetables

It's important to note that this plan is just an example, and the exact macronutrient ratios will depend on an individual's personal needs and goals. It's also important to consult with a health professional before starting any new diet or exercise plan.

My advice is to repeat this weekly plan for at least three weeks (21 days) in order to see if it works or if it needs adjustments. You can then try to switch to another carb cycling plan and see if that's better suited for you. The key number is 21, as the body and the mind need 21 days to adapt to a new reality.

It's also important to count the calories with this program, but you don't have to became obsessed by them and it's not necessary to count them every single day. You might decide to count them on a weekly basis, or even decide to restrain carbs on certain days without counting the calories. Odds are you are creating a sufficient caloric deficit, at least if you really have a decent amount of fat to lose. This can be a well strategy, at least at the beginning, it might help you start this program. If you don't have the necessary control to avoid high fat or high carb food and prefer to have things already written, it's probably best if you create a menu each week with the right amount of calories intake.

The key to have success with this plan and reach your goal is to plan ahead, if you respect the daily calories you'll soon see the results. If you also prioritize the quality of food and respect the total protein, carb and fat daily intake, then you'll see even sooner results. Adequate preparation is imperative for successful adherence to the plan; otherwise, one may find it arduous to abide by the prescribed caloric restrictions, particularly as the day progresses and one approaches the limit for caloric intake, especially in a household with other individuals or in a frenzied domestic environment. You could download a tracking calories app to help you understand how many calories you're eating and to have an idea of where you are as you go through each day.

2.7. The workout plan

Now that we've seen how carb cycling works and that we've seen some examples of how to structure a meal plan, let's remember that exercising is fundamental for this type of program. Carb cycling is often used by athletes and bodybuilders to help them reach their fitness goals. In addition to adjusting your carbohydrate intake, it's also important to adjust your workout plan. A weekly workout plan tailored to carb cycling can help you optimize your results and reach your fitness goals faster. In this section, we will provide samples of weekly workout plan for carb cycling that includes a combination of weightlifting and cardio exercises and are divided based on the difficulty level, so you can be at ease even if you don't usually workout. It is imperative to acknowledge that this regimen serves merely as a prototype and can be modified to comport with one's specific physical aptitude and aspirations. Moreover, it is crucial to heed the signals of one's physique and to regulate the plan congruently should the need arise for additional respite or an augmentation of workout intensity. Furthermore, it is indispensable to ensure adequate provision of sustenance to the body during both elevated and low carbohydrate periods. On high carb days, you should have more energy for your workouts, so you can push yourself harder and lift heavier weights. On low carb days, your energy levels may be lower, so it's important to focus on lighter weights and higher reps to maintain muscle mass.

If you are a beginner, try the beginner plan for 21 days, then switch to the intermediate one and stick to it for other 21 days. Just then you can try to switch to the expert plan.

Weekly Workout Plan (with Rest Days on Low Carb Days)

For Beginners:

Monday: High Carb Day - Strength Training (Upper Body)

Warm-up: 10 minutes of cardio (jogging, cycling, or jumping jacks)

Barbell bench press: 3 sets of 8-12 reps

Pull-ups: 3 sets of 8-12 reps

Dumbbell rows: 3 sets of 8-12 reps

Dumbbell shoulder press: 3 sets of 8-12 reps

Barbell bicep curls: 3 sets of 8-12 reps

Triceps dips: 3 sets of 8-12 reps

Cool-down: 5-10 minutes of stretching

Tuesday: Low Carb Day – Rest

Wednesday: High Carb Day - Strength Training (Lower Body)

Warm-up: 10 minutes of cardio (jogging, cycling, or jumping jacks)

Barbell squat: 3 sets of 8-12 reps

Deadlift: 3 sets of 8-12 reps

Lunges: 3 sets of 8-12 reps

Leg press: 3 sets of 8-12 reps

Calf raises: 3 sets of 8-12 reps

Cool-down: 5-10 minutes of stretching

Thursday: Low Carb Day - Rest

Friday: High Carb Day - Cardio

Warm-up: 10 minutes of cardio (jogging, cycling, or jumping jacks)

30 minutes of steady-state cardio (running, cycling, or swimming)

Cool-down: 5-10 minutes of stretching

Saturday: Low Carb Day - Rest

Sunday: High Carb Day - Cardio

Warm-up: 10 minutes of cardio (jogging, cycling, or jumping jacks)

30 minutes of steady-state cardio (running, cycling, or swimming)

Cool-down: 5-10 minutes of stretching

Intermediate:

Monday (High Carb Day):

Warm-up: 10 minutes of light cardio (jogging or cycling)

Strength Training: Full body circuit, 3 sets of 12 reps for each exercise (squats, deadlifts, bench press, rows, pull-ups, and military press)

Cardio: 30 minutes of steady-state cardio (elliptical or cycling)

Tuesday (Low Carb Day):

Yoga or stretching

Wednesday (High Carb Day):

Warm-up: 10 minutes of light cardio (jogging or cycling)

Strength Training: Upper body circuit, 3 sets of 12 reps for each exercise (push-ups, rows, pull-ups, dumbbell press, and bicep curls)

Cardio: 30 minutes of steady-state cardio (elliptical or cycling)

Thursday (Low Carb Day):

Yoga or stretching

Friday (High Carb Day):

Warm-up: 10 minutes of light cardio (jogging or cycling)

Strength Training: Lower body circuit, 3 sets of 12 reps for each exercise (squats, deadlifts, lunges, and calf raises)

Cardio: 30 minutes of steady-state cardio (elliptical or cycling)

Saturday (Low Carb Day):

Yoga or stretching

Sunday (Rest Day)

Active rest: Go for a hike or bike ride

This workout plan is designed for intermediate level fitness and includes a balance of strength training and cardio. It also includes active rest days, which are important for muscle recovery and overall health. On high carb days, the focus is on strength training and cardio, while on low carb days the focus is on yoga or stretching to promote recovery and relaxation.

For advanced:

Monday (High Carb Day):

Warm-up: 10-15 minutes of cardio (jogging, cycling, or rowing)

Strength training:

Barbell squat: 4 sets x 8-12 reps

Barbell deadlift: 4 sets x 8-12 reps

Barbell bench press: 4 sets x 8-12 reps

Pull-ups: 4 sets x 8-12 reps

Cardio: 30 minutes of high-intensity training

Cool-down: 10-15 minutes of stretching

Tuesday (Low Carb Day):

Warm-up: 10-15 minutes of cardio (jogging, cycling, or rowing)

Strength training:

Dumbbell lunges: 4 sets x 8-12 reps

Dumbbell rows: 4 sets x 8-12 reps

Dumbbell shoulder press: 4 sets x 8-12 reps

Dumbbell bicep curls: 4 sets x 8-12 reps

Cardio: 30-45 minutes of steady-state cardio (jogging, cycling, or rowing)

Cool-down: 10-15 minutes of stretching

Wednesday (High Carb Day):

Warm-up: 10-15 minutes of cardio (jogging, cycling, or rowing)

Strength training:

Barbell back squat: 4 sets x 8-12 reps

Barbell deadlift: 4 sets x 8-12 reps

Barbell bench press: 4 sets x 8-12 reps

Pull-ups: 4 sets x 8-12 reps

Cardio: 30-45 minutes of high-intensity interval training (HIIT)

Cool-down: 10-15 minutes of stretching

Thursday (Low Carb Day):

Rest day

Friday (High Carb Day):

Warm-up: 10-15 minutes of cardio (jogging, cycling, or rowing)

Strength training:

Barbell deadlift: 4 sets x 8-12 reps

Barbell squat: 4 sets x 8-12 reps

Barbell shoulder press: 4 sets x 8-12 reps

Pull-ups: 4 sets x 8-12 reps

Cardio: 30-45 minutes of high-intensity interval training (HIIT)

Cool-down: 10-15 minutes of stretching

Saturday (Low Carb Day):

Warm-up: 10-15 minutes of cardio (jogging, cycling, or rowing)

Strength training:

Dumbbell lunges: 4 sets x 8-12 reps

Dumbbell rows: 4 sets x 8-12 reps

Dumbbell shoulder press: 4 sets x 8-12 reps

Dumbbell bicep curls: 4 sets x 8-12 reps

Cardio: 30-45 minutes of steady-state cardio (jogging, cycling, or rowing)

Cool-down: 10-15 minutes of stretching

Sunday (High Carb Day):

Rest day

This workout plan is designed for intermediate to advanced individuals who are familiar with weightlifting and cardio exercises. The rest days should be adjusted accordingly, depending on the person's fitness level and goals.

2.8. Managing and tracking progress

In this chapter, we will discuss the importance of tracking progress while on a carb cycling program, as well as how to effectively manage any setbacks or challenges that may arise.

Managing and tracking progress is a crucial aspect of carb cycling. It allows you to monitor how your body is responding to the different levels of carbohydrates and make adjustments as needed. In this chapter, we will discuss the different methods of tracking progress and how to use them to optimize your carb cycling experience. This can include tracking your weight, body measurements, and progress photos, as well as keeping a food and exercise diary. Tracking your progress can also help you identify any areas where you may need to make adjustments, such as adjusting your macronutrient ratios or increasing the intensity of your workouts.

Body Measurements One of the most common ways to track progress is by taking body measurements. This includes measuring your weight, body fat percentage, and various body measurements such as your chest, waist, hips, and thighs. By taking these measurements regularly, you can see how your body is changing over time and make adjustments as needed.

Food Journaling Keeping a food journal is another great way to track progress. It allows you to see how many carbohydrates you are consuming each day and make adjustments as needed. A food journal can also help you identify any problem areas, such as overeating or eating too many processed foods.

Exercise Tracking Exercise tracking is another important aspect of carb cycling. By tracking your exercise, you can see how your body is responding to the different levels of carbohydrates and make adjustments as needed. This includes tracking the number of reps and sets you do, as well as the weight you are using.

Progress Photos Progress photos are a great way to track progress and stay motivated. By taking photos of yourself regularly, you can see how your body is changing over time and stay motivated to continue carb cycling.

Next, let's talk about managing setbacks and challenges. Carb cycling, like any diet or workout program, can be challenging at times. It's important to have a plan in place to manage any setbacks that may arise, such as a busy schedule, a lack of motivation, or a craving for high-carb foods.

One strategy to manage setbacks is to have a support system in place, such as a workout buddy or a dietitian. Another strategy is to have healthy low-carb alternatives on hand to satisfy cravings. Additionally, it can be helpful to have a plan in place for dealing with unexpected challenges, such as a last-minute business trip or a vacation.

Finally, it's important to remember that carb cycling is not a quick fix or a magic solution. It takes time and effort to see results, and it's important to be patient and persistent with your program. Remember that progress may not always be linear, and that it's normal to have setbacks and challenges along the way. With consistency and determination, however, you can achieve your goals and continue on your carb cycling journey.

In summary, managing and tracking progress is a crucial aspect of carb cycling. By using a combination of body measurements, food journaling, exercise tracking, and progress photos, you can optimize your carb cycling experience and achieve your goals. It's important to be consistent with tracking your progress, and make adjustments as necessary. Remember, the key to success with carb cycling is to find the right balance of carbohydrates that works for your body and lifestyle.

2.9. Carb cycling for long term maintenance

We've seen how carb cycling works and what the benefits are. It is imperative to comprehend that carb cycling is not merely a facile method for shedding weight, but rather a comprehensive approach. It's a life style that will forever change your eating habits. It is feasible to continue carb cycling after attaining one's weight objective, albeit with some modifications to the plan. This approach can sustain a desired weight and optimize the body's fat-metabolizing proficiency to ensure they remain at optimal performance levels.

Adhering to the following fundamental tenets of carb cycling is critical:

1. Consuming breakfast on a daily basis.

2. Engaging in five meals per day, commencing with a breakfast meal within thirty minutes of awakening, and subsequent meals every three hours.

3. Follow your program.

These are not difficult rules, but they can be tricky depending on the lifestyle of each person. Especially the "eat breakfast every day" rule and the "eat 5 times a day" rule can be a bit of an obstacle if you're not used to such lifestyle. Especially at the beginning. Since we are constantly surrounded by poor diet foods and are pushed by the society to skip meals, or we don't have time to actually prepare them, these simple three rules appear incredibly difficult.

Thus, it is imperative that, in addition to adhering to the fundamental tenets of carb cycling, individuals cultivate the capability to make astute selections with regards to their alimentary and lifestyle practices. Fast food establishments are commonly recognized as purveyors of unhealthful fare, characterized by their high levels of lipid, grease, and oil. However, in many instances, these establishments offer menu items that can be reconciled with a carb cycling diet. For instance, baked potatoes can be a suitable snack, while salads are frequently available as well. If consuming a sandwich, opt for ingredients that are more nutritious and less fatty, such as lean meats like turkey, or select seafood options such as tuna or salmon. Furthermore, one can eliminate small additions, such as mayonnaise, salad dressings, and certain nuts or fruits that are overly rich in fat and sugar.

Carb cycling is a matter of mastery, where one wields control over the metabolic processes of one's physique and the choices that one makes. These are transformations in lifestyle that must be internalized and sustained for the long term, potentially for a lifetime. It is vital to remain steadfast in one's adherence to the program and to continually keep one's goals in clear focus.

PART THREE

EASY RECIPES

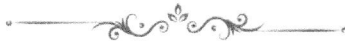

3.1. BREAKFAST

HIGH CARB DAY BREAKFAST

Oatmeal with Berries and Protein Powder (2 servings) – 10 minutes

Ingredients:

- 2 cups rolled oats
- 2 cups almond milk
- 1 cup mixed berries
- 2 scoops vanilla protein powder
- 2 tbsp honey (optional)

Procedure:

- In a medium-sized pot, bring 2 cups of water to a boil.
- Add 1 cup of rolled oats and reduce heat to low.
- Let simmer for 5 minutes or until oats are cooked through.

- Remove from heat and agitate with 2 portions of vanilla-flavoured protein powder and 2 teaspoons of honey.

- Divide the oatmeal into 2 bowls.

- In a small saucepan, combine 1/2 cup of frozen berries with 1/4 cup of water.

- Heat over medium heat until the berries are thawed, and the mixture is hot.

- Divide the berry mixture over the oatmeal in each bowl.

- Serve warm and enjoy.

The oatmeal provides a good source of carbohydrates, while the protein powder and berries add a boost of protein. you can switch up the type of berries, or even add nuts or seeds for extra crunch and flavour. Also, if you prefer a sweeter taste, you can add more honey or any sweetener that you like.

Macros x serving

Calories: 300   Protein: 25g   Carbohydrates: 35g   Fat: 6g

Greek Yogurt with Berries and Granola (2 servings) – 5 minutes

Ingredients:

- 2 cups Greek yogurt

- 1 cup mixed berries

- 1/2 cup granola

- 2 tbsp honey (optional)

Procedure:

- In a medium-sized mixing bowl, combine 2 cups of Greek yogurt.

- Divide the yogurt into 2 bowls.

- In a small saucepan, combine 1 cup of frozen berries with 1/4 cup of water.

- Heat over medium heat until the berries are thawed, and the mixture is hot.

- Divide the berry mixture over the Greek yogurt in each bowl.

- Add 1/4 cup of granola over each bowl of yogurt and berries.

- Serve and enjoy.

This dish serves as a commendable breakfast alternative, boasting a harmonious balance of protein and carbohydrates. The Greek yogurt provides a substantial dose of protein, complemented by the assimilation of antioxidants and flavour through the addition of berries. The granola provides a nice crunch and extra carbs. You can switch up the type of berries or granola to keep it interesting. If you prefer a sweeter taste, you can add more honey or any sweetener that you like.

Macros x serving

Calories: 250   Protein: 20g   Carbohydrates: 25g   Fat: 5g

Blueberry Banana Protein Smoothie (2 servings) – 5 minutes

Ingredients:

- 1 banana

- 1 cup frozen blueberries

- 2 scoops vanilla protein powder

- 2 cups almond milk

- 2 tsp honey

Procedure:

- In a blender, combine 1 banana, 1 cup frozen blueberries, 2 scoops of vanilla protein powder, 2 cups of almond milk, and 2 tsp of honey.

- Blend until smooth.

- Divide the smoothie into 2 servings and enjoy.

This recipe is a great option for a high-carb, high-protein breakfast. The banana and blueberries provide carbohydrates, while the protein powder and almond milk add a boost of protein. This smoothie is easy to make and can be taken on the go, perfect for busy mornings. Feel free to experiment with different types of berries, or even add spinach or kale to increase the nutrient content. If you prefer a sweeter taste, you can add more honey or any sweetener that you like.

Macros x serving

Calories: 250   Protein: 20g   Carbohydrates: 30g   Fat: 5g

Peanut Butter Banana Oatmeal (2 servings) – 10 minutes

Ingredients:

- 1 cup rolled oats
- 2 banana
- 2 tbsp peanut butter
- 2 cups almond milk
- 2 tsp honey

Procedure:

- In a medium-sized pot, bring 2 cups of water to a boil.
- Add 1 cup of rolled oats and reduce heat to low.
- Let simmer for 5 minutes or until oats are cooked through.
- Remove from heat and stir in 2 tbsp of peanut butter and 2 tsp of honey.
- Divide the oatmeal into 2 bowls.
- Cut 2 bananas into small slices, divide the banana slices over the oatmeal in each bowl.
- Serve warm and enjoy.

This recipe is a great option for those who are looking for a high-carb, high-protein breakfast. The oatmeal constitutes a commendable origin of carbohydrates, while the inclusion of peanut butter and banana elevates the protein content and imparts an enhancement of flavour. You can switch up the type of nut butter, or even add nuts or seeds for extra crunch and flavour. Also, if you prefer a sweeter taste, you can add more honey or any sweetener that you like.

Macros x serving

Calories: 300 Protein: 10g   Carbohydrates: 35g   Fat: 12g

Banana Pancakes (2 servings) – 20 minutes

Ingredients:

- 2 bananas

- 4 eggs

- 1/2 cup whole wheat flour

- 1/2 tsp baking powder

- 2 tsp honey

Procedure:

- In a large mixing bowl, mash 2 bananas with a fork or potato masher.

- Whisk in 4 eggs, 1/2 cup of whole wheat flour and 1/2 tsp of baking powder.

- Heat a skillet over medium-high heat, add a little butter or oil.

- Using a ladle, pour batter onto skillet, cook until the surface of pancakes have some bubbles, then flip carefully with a spatula, and cook until golden brown.

- Proceed until the mixture has been exhausted.

- Serve with 2 tsp of honey on top and divide into two servings.

This recipe is simple, easy, and delicious. The ripe bananas add natural sweetness and flavour to the pancakes, and the eggs and flour provide structure and protein. You can add some cinnamon or vanilla extract for extra flavour. You can also make these gluten-free by using a gluten-free flour blend instead of all-purpose flour. And if you prefer a lower calorie option, you can use a non-stick cooking spray instead of butter or oil.

Macros x serving

Calories: 250   Protein: 10g   Carbohydrates: 25g   Fat: 10g

Blueberry Muffins (2 servings) – 30 minutes

Ingredients:

- 1/2 cup whole wheat flour
- 1/2 cup oat flour
- 1/4 tsp baking powder
- 1/4 tsp baking soda
- 1/4 cup honey
- 1 egg
- 1/4 cup Greek yogurt
- 1/4 cup blueberries

Procedure:

- Preheat your oven to 350°F (175°C).
- In a medium-sized mixing bowl, combine 1 cup of whole

wheat flour, 1 cup of oat flour, 1/2 tsp baking powder, and 1/2 tsp baking soda.

- In a separate mixing bowl, whisk 1/2 cup honey, 2 eggs, and 1/2 cup of Greek yogurt.

- With a delicate touch, incorporate the moist components into the arid constituents until they are merely amalgamated.

- Stir in 1/2 cup of blueberries.

- Divide batter into a greased muffin tin or lined with muffin cups.

- Bake in preheated oven for 20-25 minutes or until a toothpick inserted into the centre of a muffin comes out clean.

- Let cool in the pan for 5 minutes before removing them to a wire rack to cool completely.

This recipe is a delicious way to start your day, blueberry muffins are a classic breakfast treat. These muffins embody a harmonious fusion of saccharine and acidulous flavours, enshrouded with salubrious elements such as whole wheat flour, oat flour, Greek yogurt, and blueberries. Their preparation is elementary, and you can even prepare a large quantity beforehand, preserving them in the freezer for expeditious morning sustenance. You can also switch up the type of berries, or even add nuts or seeds for extra crunch and flavour. If you prefer a sweeter taste, you can add more honey or any sweetener that you like.

Macros x serving

Calories: 250   Protein: 8g   Carbohydrates: 35g   Fat: 10g

LOW CARB DAY BREAKFAST

Egg and Sausage Breakfast Bowl (2 servings) – 15 minutes

Ingredients:

- 4 eggs
- 4 turkey sausages
- 1 cup diced bell pepper
- 1/2 cup diced onion
- 2 tbsp olive oil
- Salt and pepper to taste

Procedure:

- Heat a skillet over medium-high heat, add a tablespoon of olive oil.
- Add 8 oz of diced turkey or pork sausage to the skillet, cook until browned, about 5-7 minutes.
- Remove the sausage from the skillet and set it aside.
- Crack 4 eggs into the skillet and scramble until cooked through, about 3-5 minutes.
- Remove the eggs from the skillet and set them aside.
- In the same skillet, add 1/2 cup diced bell pepper and 1/2 cup diced onion, sauté until they are tender.
- Add the cooked sausage and eggs to the skillet with the vegetables, stir to combine.

- Divide the mixture into 2 servings and enjoy.

This recipe is a great option for those who are looking for a high-protein, low-carb breakfast. You can add more veggies or seasonings to suit your taste and you can also switch up the type of sausage you use to keep it interesting. If you prefer to make it more keto-friendly, you can serve it in a bowl without the carbs of rice or quinoa.

Macros x serving

Calories: 300   Protein: 20g   Carbohydrates: 7g   Fat: 20g

Breakfast Scramble with Spinach and Feta (2 servings) – 10 minutes

Ingredients:

- 4 eggs
- 1/2 cup diced onion
- 2 cups spinach
- 4 tbsp crumbled feta cheese
- Salt and pepper to taste

Procedure:

- Heat a skillet over medium heat, add a tablespoon of olive oil.
- Crack 4 eggs into a mixing bowl, add 2 tbsp of milk and beat until well combined.
- Add 1/2 cup diced onion and 1 cup of spinach to the skillet

and sauté until the onion is translucent and the spinach is wilted.

- Pour the eggs into the skillet, stir occasionally until the eggs are cooked through.

- Remove from heat and stir in 4 tbsp of crumbled feta cheese.

- Divide into 2 servings and enjoy.

This recipe is quite easy and simple to make, it's a combination of healthy greens, eggs, and cheese, which makes it a perfect low-carb breakfast option. You can add more veggies or even diced meats to this scramble to make it more flavourful and filling.

Macros x serving

Calories: 150   Protein: 12g   Carbohydrates: 2g   Fat: 12g

Breakfast Avocado Toast (2 servings) – 5 minutes

Ingredients:

- 4 slices whole wheat bread

- 2 avocados

- 4 boiled eggs

- Salt and pepper to taste

Procedure:

- Toast 4 slices of whole wheat bread to desired level of doneness.

- Cut avocado in half and remove the pit, then mash the avocado in a small bowl.

- Spread mashed avocado onto toasted bread slices.

- Slice two boiled eggs and place on top of the mashed avocado.

- Season with salt and pepper to taste.

This recipe is a simple, easy, and delicious breakfast option. The avocado provides healthy fats, and the eggs provide protein. The whole wheat bread provides complex carbohydrates and fibre. This recipe is easy to customize, you can add other veggies, herbs, or cheese to give it a different flavour or you can switch up the type of bread.

Macros x serving

Calories: 400   Protein: 15g   Carbohydrates: 30g   Fat: 25g

Breakfast Frittata with vegetables (2 servings) – 15 minutes

Ingredients:

- 6 eggs
- 1/2 cup diced bell pepper
- 1/2 cup diced onion
- 1/2 cup diced mushrooms
- Salt and pepper to taste
- 4 tbsp grated Parmesan cheese

Procedure:

- Preheat oven to 350°F (175°C).

- Whisk 6 eggs in a mixing bowl, add salt and pepper to taste.

- Heat 2 tbsp of oil in a skillet over medium-high heat.

- Add diced onion, diced bell pepper, and diced mushrooms to the skillet.

- Sauté for 5 minutes, or until vegetables are tender.

- Pour whisked eggs into skillet and stir gently.

- Sprinkle 4 tbsp of grated Parmesan cheese over the top.

- Bake in preheated oven for 8-10 minutes, or until the frittata is set and golden on top.

- Let cool for a few minutes before slicing and serving.

This recipe is a perfect low-carb breakfast option. It's packed with vegetables, eggs, and cheese, which makes it a delicious and healthy way to start your day. You can add other vegetables or even diced meats to this frittata to make it more flavourful and filling. Additionally, you can also add some herbs or spices to give it a different flavour.

Macros x serving

Calories: 200   Protein: 15g   Carbohydrates: 3g   Fat: 15g

Breakfast Burrito with Spinach and Feta (2 servings) – 10 minutes

Ingredients:

- 2 eggs

- 1/4 cup diced onion

- 1 cup spinach

- 2 tbsp crumbled feta cheese

- 2 tbsp salsa

- Salt and pepper to taste

- 2 tbsp avocado

Procedure:

- Crack 4 eggs into a mixing bowl, whisk and season with salt and pepper.

- Heat a skillet over medium heat, add 1/2 cup diced onion and 1 cup spinach.

- Cook until the onion is translucent, and the spinach is wilted.

- Pour the whisked eggs over the vegetables and stir occasionally until the eggs are cooked.

- Remove from heat and stir in 4 tbsp of crumbled feta cheese.

- Warm up 4 tbsp of salsa in the microwave for a few seconds.

- Place a 1/2 cup of the egg and vegetable mixture on each of the 4 tortillas.

- Spread 2 tbsp of warmed salsa on top of each tortilla.

- Top each tortilla with 2 tbsp of diced avocado and roll them up tightly.

- Serve warm and enjoy.

This repast is a scrumptious and effortless mode of initiating one's day and is also suitable for those in search of a low-carb breakfast. The eggs, spinach, and feta cheese furnish a substantial amount of protein, while the salsa and avocado impart an enhancement of taste and salubrious lipids. You can add other veggies or seasonings to suit your taste and you can also switch up the type of cheese you use to keep it interesting.

Macros x serving

Calories: 250   Protein: 15g   Carbohydrates: 10g   Fat: 20g

Breakfast Omelette with Spinach and Tomato (2 servings) – 15 minutes

Ingredients:

- 2 eggs
- 1/4 cup diced spinach
- 1/4 cup diced tomato
- 1/4 cup diced mushrooms
- Salt and pepper to taste
- 2 tbsp grated Parmesan cheese

Procedure:

- In a mixing bowl, whisk 2 eggs and season with salt and pepper.
- Heat a skillet over medium heat, add 1/4 cup diced spinach, 1/4 cup diced tomato, 1/4 cup diced mushrooms.

- Cook until vegetables are tender.

- Pour whisked eggs over the vegetables and stir occasionally until the eggs are cooked.

- Sprinkle 2 tbsp grated Parmesan cheese over the top.

- Carefully fold the omelette in half and slide it onto a plate.

- Serve warm and enjoy.

This recipe is a great low-carb breakfast option, it's packed with protein, veggies, and cheese. It's also very versatile, you can add other vegetables or meats to this omelette to make it more flavourful and filling. You can also switch up the type of cheese you use to keep it interesting. You can also add herbs or spices to give it a different flavour.

Macros x serving

Calories: 150   Protein: 12g   Carbohydrates: 3g   Fat: 12g

3.2. LUNCH

HIGH CARB DAY LUNCH

Whole Wheat Pita with Falafel and Tzatziki Sauce (2 servings) – 30 minutes

Ingredients:

- 2 whole wheat pita bread
- 4 falafel balls

- 1/4 cup tzatziki sauce

- 1/4 cup diced cucumber

- 1/4 cup diced tomatoes

- 1/4 cup diced red onion

- Salt and pepper to taste

Procedure:

- Preheat oven to 350°F (175°C).

- Place the falafel balls on a baking sheet and bake for 10-15 minutes, or until golden brown and crispy.

- While the falafel is baking, prepare the tzatziki sauce by mixing together 1/2 cup of plain Greek yogurt, 1/4 cup of diced cucumber, 1 tablespoon of chopped fresh dill, 1 tablespoon of lemon juice, and salt and pepper to taste in a small mixing bowl.

- Warm the pita bread in the oven for a few minutes or in a skillet over medium heat.

- Cut the pita bread in half and fill with falafel balls, diced tomatoes, red onion, and tzatziki sauce.

- Serve and enjoy.

This recipe is a delicious and healthy Middle Eastern dish. The whole wheat pita bread provides complex carbohydrates, while the falafel and tzatziki sauce provide protein and healthy fats. You can add more veggies or greens such as lettuce, parsley, or mint, or even switch up the type of bread. You can also adjust the amount of tzatziki sauce according to your taste preference.

Macros x serving

Calories: 300   Protein: 12g   Carbohydrates: 40g   Fat:15g

～❉～

Whole Wheat Pasta with Meatballs and Marinara Sauce (2 servings) – 25 minutes

Ingredients:

- 8 oz whole wheat pasta
- 8 beef or pork meatballs
- 1 cup marinara sauce
- 2 tbsp grated Parmesan cheese
- Salt and pepper to taste

Procedure:

- Cook pasta according to package instructions. Drain and set aside.
- In a skillet over medium-high heat, cook the meatballs for 10-12 minutes or until cooked through.
- Add the marinara sauce to the skillet and stir to coat the meatballs.
- Cook for an additional 2-3 minutes, or until the sauce is heated through.
- Divide the pasta into two servings, top each with half of the meatballs and marinara sauce, and sprinkle with grated Parmesan cheese.
- Serve and enjoy.

This recipe is a delicious and easy way to enjoy a pasta dish. The whole wheat pasta provides complex carbohydrates, while the meatballs and marinara sauce provide a good source of protein. You can add more veggies such as bell pepper, mushrooms, or zucchini to increase the volume of the dish and make it more filling. You can also adjust the amount of cheese and sauce according to your taste preference.

Macros per serving

Calories: 400   Protein: 25g   Carbohydrates: 40g   Fat: 15g

Grilled Vegetable and Quinoa Salad (2 servings) – 30 minutes

Ingredients:

- 1/2 cup quinoa
- 1/2 cup vegetable broth
- 1 red bell pepper, sliced
- 1 yellow bell pepper, sliced
- 1 zucchini, sliced
- 1 red onion, sliced
- 2 tbsp olive oil
- 1 tsp balsamic vinegar
- Salt and pepper to taste

Procedure:

- Cook the quinoa according to package instructions, using

vegetable broth instead of water. Let it cool.

- Warm up a grill or grill pan over medium heat.

- In a large bowl, toss together the sliced bell peppers, zucchini, and red onion with olive oil, balsamic vinegar, salt and pepper.

- Grill the vegetables for about 5-7 minutes per side or until tender and charred.

- In a large bowl, combine the cooked quinoa and grilled vegetables.

- Divide the salad into two servings and serve.

This Grilled Vegetable and Quinoa Salad is a high-carb recipe that you can have as a lunch option on your carb cycling diet. It constitutes a nutritious and delectable alternative that is uncomplicated to prepare and replete with nourishing elements. It is an efficacious manner of obtaining one's quotidian intake of vegetables and integral cereals, yet still preserving a substantial carbohydrate content.

Macros per serving

Calories: 350   Protein: 8g   Carbohydrates: 40g   Fat: 18g

Whole Wheat Wrap with Hummus, Vegetables and Feta Cheese (2 servings) – 15 minutes

Ingredients:

- 2 whole wheat wraps

- 1/4 cup hummus

- 1/4 cup diced tomatoes

- 1/4 cup diced cucumber
- 1/4 cup diced bell pepper
- 2 tbsp crumbled feta cheese
- Salt and pepper to taste

Procedure:

- Spread hummus over the wraps, leaving a 1/2-inch border around the edges.

- Add the diced vegetables and crumbled feta cheese over the hummus.

- Season with salt and pepper.

- Roll up the wraps tightly and cut in half diagonally.

- Serve and enjoy!

This Whole Wheat Wrap with Hummus, Vegetables, and Feta Cheese is a high-carb recipe that can be enjoyed as a lunch option on your carb cycling diet. The utilization of whole wheat wraps as a base affords a viable source of complex carbohydrates, while the combination of hummus, vegetables, and feta cheese constitutes a judicious balance of proteins, salubrious fats, and essential micronutrients. The recipe is easy to make and can be prepared in advance, making it a convenient option for busy days.

Macros per serving

Calories: 300   Protein: 8g   Carbohydrates: 40g   Fat: 12g

Grilled Steak with Roasted Potatoes and Carrots (2 servings) – 30 minutes

Ingredients:

- 2 (8 oz) sirloin steaks
- 1 lb baby potatoes, halved
- 1 lb carrots, peeled and cut into 2-inch pieces
- 2 tbsp olive oil
- Salt and pepper to taste

Procedure:

- Preheat oven to 425°F (220°C).
- Toss the potatoes and carrots in olive oil, salt, and pepper. Spread the vegetables on a baking sheet and bake for 25-30 minutes.
- Heat a skillet over medium-high heat.
- Season the steaks with salt and pepper.
- Grill the steaks for 3-4 minutes per side for medium-rare, or longer if desired.
- Remove the steaks from the skillet and let them rest for 5 minutes.
- Serve the steaks with the roasted potatoes and carrots.
- Serve and enjoy.

This Grilled Steak with Roasted Potatoes and Carrots is a high-carb recipe that can be enjoyed as a lunch option on your carb cycling diet. The potatoes and carrots provide a good source of complex carbohydrates, while the steak provides a good source of protein. This recipe is easy to make and can be prepared in advance, making it a convenient option for busy days.

Macros per serving

Calories: 500   Protein: 25g   Carbohydrates: 50g   Fat: 20g

Whole Wheat Pizza with Vegetables and Mozzarella (2 servings) – 20 minutes

Ingredients:

- 2 whole wheat pizza crusts
- 1/2 cup marinara sauce
- 1/2 cup sliced mushrooms
- 1/2 cup sliced bell peppers
- 1/2 cup sliced onions
- 1 cup shredded mozzarella cheese
- Salt and pepper to taste

Procedure:

- Preheat oven to 425°F (220°C).
- Place the pizza crusts on a baking sheet or pizza pan.
- Spread marinara sauce over the crusts, leaving a 1/2-inch

border around the edges.

- Top with sliced mushrooms, bell peppers, and onions.

- Sprinkle with mozzarella cheese and season with salt and pepper.

- Bake for 12-15 minutes or until the crust is golden brown and the cheese is melted.

- Serve and enjoy.

This Whole Wheat Pizza with Vegetables and Mozzarella is a high-carb recipe that can be enjoyed as a lunch option on your carb cycling diet. The pizza base fashioned from whole wheat flour and the presence of vegetables afford a substantial measure of complex carbohydrates, while the cheese and the animal protein provide a substantial amount of protein. This recipe is easy to make and can be prepared in advance, making it a convenient option for busy days. You can also adjust the vegetables you like and add other toppings as you please.

Macros per serving

Calories: 500   Protein: 20g   Carbohydrates: 50g   Fat: 20g

Whole Wheat Pasta with Pesto, Tomatoes, and Mozzarella (2 servings) – 20 minutes

Ingredients:

- 8 oz whole wheat pasta

- 1/2 cup basil pesto

- 1 cup cherry tomatoes, halved

- 1/2 cup shredded mozzarella cheese
- Salt and pepper to taste

Procedure:

- Boil a large pot of water. Add the pasta and cook about 8-10 minutes. Drain and set aside.

- In a large mixing bowl, add the pesto, tomatoes, and mozzarella cheese. Toss to combine.

- Add the cooked pasta to the pesto mixture and toss again until the pasta is evenly coated.

- Add salt and pepper to taste.

- Serve warm.

This recipe contains a balance of macronutrients, including high-quality carbohydrates from the whole wheat pasta and healthy fats from the pesto and mozzarella. Additionally, the serving size is easily adjustable to fit your individual needs for the day, making it a versatile option for carb cycling.

Macros per serving

Calories: 550   Protein: 20g   Carbohydrates: 84g   Fat: 18g

LOW CARB DAY LUNCH:

Grilled Chicken Caesar Salad – 25 minutes

Ingredients:

- 2 boneless, skinless chicken breasts

- 2 cups chopped romaine lettuce

- 2 tbsp Caesar dressing

- 2 tbsp grated Parmesan cheese

- 2 tbsp croutons

- Salt and pepper to taste

Procedure:

- Preheat a grill or grill pan.

- Add salt and pepper.

- Grill the chicken for 6-7 minutes per side, or until cooked through.

- Remove the chicken from the grill and let it rest for 5 minutes before slicing.

- In a large bowl, toss together the romaine lettuce, Caesar dressing, grated Parmesan cheese, and croutons.

- Divide the salad into two servings, top each with half of the sliced chicken.

- Serve and enjoy.

This recipe is a delicious and healthy way to enjoy a Caesar salad. The succulent grilled chicken serves as a substantial source of protein, while the crisp lettuce and the flavourful dressing offer a rich source of vital vitamins and minerals. You can add more veggies or greens such as tomatoes, cucumber, or bell pepper to increase the volume of the salad and make it more filling. You can also adjust the amount of dressing and cheese according to your taste preference.

Macros per serving

Calories: 300   Protein: 30g   Carbohydrates: 12g   Fat: 20g

Grilled Salmon with Mixed Greens (2 servings) - 25 minutes

Ingredients:

- 2 (4 oz) salmon fillets
- 2 cups mixed greens
- 2 tbsp vinaigrette dressing
- Salt and pepper to taste

Procedure:

- Preheat grill to medium-high heat.
- Add salt and pepper to the salmon fillets.
- Grill the salmon for 4-5 minutes per side, or until cooked through.
- In a large bowl, toss together the mixed greens with vinaigrette dressing.
- Divide the mixed greens into two servings, top each with a grilled salmon fillet.
- Serve and enjoy

This recipe is a delicious and healthy way to enjoy a salmon dish. The grilled salmon presents a commendable source of protein and salubrious omega-3 lipids, while the heterogeneous greens furnish an advantageous quantity of vitamins and minerals. You can also switch up the type of greens, add other veggies, or even switch up the type of dressing to give it a different flavour.

Macros per serving

Calories: 250   Protein: 25g   Carbohydrates: 5g   Fat: 15g

Grilled Chicken Salad (2 servings) – 25 minutes

Ingredients:

- 2 boneless, skinless chicken breasts
- 2 cups mixed greens
- 2 tbsp vinaigrette dressing
- 1/4 cup diced cucumber
- 1/4 cup diced tomatoes
- 1/4 cup diced red onion
- Salt and pepper to taste

Procedure:

- Preheat grill or grill pan.
- Add salt or pepper to the chicken breasts.
- Grill the chicken for 6-7 minutes per side, or until cooked through.

- Remove the chicken from the grill and let it rest for 5 minutes before slicing.

- In a large bowl, toss together the mixed greens, vinaigrette dressing, diced cucumber, diced tomatoes, and diced red onion.

- Divide the salad into two servings, top each with half of the sliced chicken.

- Serve and enjoy!

This recipe is a delicious and healthy way to enjoy a chicken salad dish. You can also switch up the type of greens, add other veggies, or even switch up the type of dressing to give it a different flavour.

Macros per serving

Calories: 200   Protein: 25g   Carbohydrates: 5g   Fat: 10g

Grilled Steak with Broccoli (2 servings) – 25 minutes

Ingredients:

- 2 (4 oz) boneless beef steaks
- 2 cups broccoli florets
- 2 tbsp olive oil
- 1/2 tsp garlic powder
- Salt and pepper to taste

Procedure:

- Preheat grill or grill pan..

- Season the steaks with garlic powder, salt, and pepper.

- Grill the steaks for 4-5 minutes per side, or until cooked to desired doneness.

- While the steaks are cooking, in a separate pan, sauté the broccoli florets in olive oil for 5-7 minutes or until tender.

- Divide the broccoli into two servings, top each with a grilled steak.

- Serve and enjoy!

This recipe is a delicious and healthy way to enjoy a steak dish. The grilled steak provides a good source of protein, while the broccoli provides a good source of vitamins and minerals. You can also switch up the side dish, add other veggies, or even switch up the seasonings to give it a different flavour.

Macros per serving

Calories: 300   Protein: 25g   Carbohydrates: 5g   Fat: 25g

Chicken and Vegetable Stir Fry (2 servings) – 25 minutes

Ingredients:

- 2 boneless, skinless chicken breasts, sliced

- 1 cup sliced bell peppers

- 1 cup sliced mushrooms

- 1 cup sliced onion

- 2 tbsp olive oil

- 2 cloves garlic, minced

- 2 tbsp soy sauce

- Salt and pepper to taste

Procedure:

- Warm up a large pan.

- Add the olive oil, garlic, and chicken. Cook for 5-7 minutes, check the chicken to see if it's cooked before taking it from the pan.

- Add the bell peppers, mushrooms, and onion. Cook for an additional 5-7 minutes, check if the vegetables are tender before taking them out of the pan.

- Stir in the soy sauce and cook for an additional 1-2 minutes.

- Season with salt and pepper.

- Divide the stir fry into two servings and serve.

This Chicken and Vegetable Stir Fry is a low-carb recipe that can be enjoyed as a lunch option on your carb cycling diet. The poultry serves as a rich repository of protean sustenance, whilst the leguminous and nutrient-rich edibles serve to supply a copious quantity of dietary fibre and nourishment. The brown rice can be added as an option for high carb day. This recipe is easy to make and can be prepared in advance, making it a convenient option for busy days. You can also adjust the vegetables you like and add other toppings as you please.

Macros per serving

Calories: 250   Protein: 25g   Carbohydrates: 5g   Fat: 15g

***

Tuna Salad Lettuce Wraps (2 servings) – 15 minutes

Ingredients:

- 2 cans tuna, drained
- 2 tbsp mayonnaise
- 1 tbsp Dijon mustard
- 1/4 cup diced celery
- 1/4 cup diced onion
- Salt and pepper to taste
- 4 lettuce leaves

Procedure:

- In a medium-sized bowl, mix together the tuna, mayonnaise, Dijon mustard, celery, and onion.
- Add salt and pepper to taste.
- Lay out the lettuce leaves on a plate.
- Divide the tuna salad mixture into two portions and spoon it onto the centre of each lettuce leaf.
- Fold the lettuce leaf around the tuna mixture to form a wrap.
- Serve and enjoy.

This Tuna Salad Lettuce Wraps recipe is a low-carb recipe that can be enjoyed as a lunch option on your carb cycling diet. The Tuna supplies a commendable quantity of protein and wholesome omega-3 fatty acids, whilst the lettuce offers a satisfactory provision of fibre and micronutrients. This recipe is easy to make and can be prepared in advance, making it a convenient option for busy days. You can also adjust the ingredients you like and add other toppings as you please.

Macros per serving

Calories: 250   Protein: 25g   Carbohydrates: 5g   Fat: 15g

Cabbage and Sausage Stir Fry (2 servings) – 30 minutes

Ingredients:

- 8 oz turkey sausage, sliced
- 2 cups shredded cabbage
- 1/2 cup diced onion
- 1/2 cup diced bell pepper
- 1 tbsp olive oil
- Salt and pepper to taste

Procedure:

- Warm up a large pan over medium-heat and add the olive oil.
- Add the turkey sausage and cook for about 3-4 minutes, until browned.
- Add the onion, bell pepper, and cabbage to the skillet and stir-fry for about 5 minutes, until the vegetables are tender.
- Add with salt and pepper to taste.

- Serve immediately.

This recipe is optimal for low carbohydrate dietary regimens due to its moderate proportion of carbohydrates and elevated concentration of protein. The vegetables provide fibre and nutrients, and the turkey sausage adds flavour and satiety. The stir-fry method of cooking is quick and easy, making it a convenient option for busy individuals.

Macros per serving

Calories: 150   Protein: 14g   Carbohydrates: 4g   Fat: 10g

3.3. DINNER

HIGH CARB DAY DINNER:

Baked Chicken Parmesan (2 servings) - 30 minutes

Ingredients:

- 2 boneless, skinless chicken breasts
- 1/2 cup Italian-seasoned breadcrumbs
- 1/4 cup grated Parmesan cheese
- 1 egg
- 1/4 cup all-purpose flour
- 1/2 cup marinara sauce
- 1 cup shredded mozzarella cheese

- Salt and pepper to taste

Procedure:

- Preheat oven to 375°F (190°C).

- In a shallow dish, combine the breadcrumbs and Parmesan cheese.

- In another shallow dish, beat the egg.

- Place the flour in a third shallow dish.

- Add salt and pepper.

- Dredge the chicken breasts in the flour, then dip in the beaten egg, and finally coat in the breadcrumb mixture.

- Place the chicken in a baking dish and top with marinara sauce and shredded mozzarella cheese.

- Bake for 25-30 minutes or until the chicken is cooked through and the cheese is golden brown.

- Serve and enjoy.

You can also serve this dish with a side of whole wheat spaghetti or a side salad to increase the carb content even more.

Macros per serving

Calories: 500   Protein: 30g   Carbohydrates: 30g   Fat: 25g

Grilled Salmon with Quinoa and Asparagus (2 servings) – 20 minutes

Ingredients:

- 2 (6 oz) salmon fillets

- 2 tbsp olive oil

- Salt and pepper to taste

- 2 cups cooked quinoa

- 1 bunch asparagus, trimmed

Procedure:

- Heat a grill or grill pan a medium to high thermal intensity.

- Add with salt and pepper and oil.

- Grill the salmon for 4-5 minutes per side or until cooked through.

- In a separate pan, sauté the asparagus in olive oil and season with salt and pepper. Cook for 2-3 minutes.

- Serve the grilled salmon with the quinoa and sautéed asparagus and enjoy.

You can also add some sliced lemon on top of the fish for some extra taste.

Macros per serving

Calories: 550   Protein: 35g   Carbohydrates: 40g   Fat: 25g

Whole Wheat Penne with Meat Sauce (2 servings) – 30 minutes

Ingredients:

- 8 oz whole wheat penne pasta

- 1 lb ground beef

- 1 onion, diced

- 2 cloves garlic, minced

- 1 () can diced tomatoes

- 1/2 cup beef broth

- 1 tbsp tomato paste

- 2 tsp dried oregano

- 1 tsp dried basil

- Salt and pepper to taste

- 1/4 cup grated Parmesan cheese

Procedure:

- Cook the pasta. Drain and set aside.

- In a large skillet, brown the ground beef over medium-high heat. Drain any excess fat.

- Add the onion and garlic to the skillet and sauté for 2-3 minutes or until softened.

- Add the diced tomatoes, beef broth, tomato paste, oregano, basil, salt, and pepper. Stir to combine.

- Bring the mixture to a simmer and let it cook for 10-15 minutes or until the sauce thickens.

- Add it in the cooked pasta and grated Parmesan.

- Serve and enjoy.

You can also add some vegetables like mushrooms, peppers, or zucchini to increase the nutritional value of the dish.

Macros per serving

Calories: 600   Protein: 30g   Carbohydrates: 75g   Fat: 20g

Chicken and Vegetable Fried Rice (2 servings) – 25 minutes

Ingredients:

- 2 cups cooked brown rice
- 1 lb boneless, skinless chicken breast, diced
- 1 tbsp vegetable oil
- 2 cloves garlic, minced
- 1/2 onion, diced
- 1/2 cup frozen peas
- 1/2 cup frozen carrots
- 2 tbsp soy sauce
- 2 green onions, thinly sliced

Procedure:

- In a big pan, heat the vegetable oil.
- Add the chicken and stir fry for 3-4 minutes or until cooked through. Remove from skillet and set aside. 3. In the same skillet, add garlic and onion and sauté for 2-3 minutes until softened.
- Add the frozen peas and carrots and continue to sauté for another 2-3 minutes until the vegetables are tender.

- Stir in the cooked brown rice, soy sauce, and green onions. Cook for 2-3 minutes.

- Add the cooked chicken back into the skillet and stir to combine.

- Serve and enjoy.

You can also add some more vegetables or different proteins like shrimp or tofu to make it more diverse.

Macros per serving

Calories: 550   Protein: 30g   Carbohydrates: 75g   Fat: 15g

Whole Wheat Pasta with Meatballs and Marinara Sauce (2 servings) – 30 minutes

Ingredients:

- 8 oz whole wheat pasta

- 1 lb ground beef

- 1 egg

- 1/4 cup breadcrumbs

- 1/4 cup grated Parmesan cheese

- 2 cloves garlic, minced

- 1/4 cup chopped fresh parsley

- Salt and pepper to taste

- 1 (24 oz) jar marinara sauce

- 1/4 cup grated mozzarella cheese

Procedure:

- Cook the pasta. Drain and set aside.

- In a mixing bowl, combine ground beef, egg, breadcrumbs, Parmesan cheese, garlic, parsley, salt, and pepper. Mix well.

- Roll the mixture into 1-inch meatballs.

- In a large skillet, brown the meatballs over medium-high heat for 8-10 minutes, or until cooked through.

- Add the marinara sauce and stir to coat the meatballs.

- Add the cooked pasta and mix with the sauce.

- Sprinkle mozzarella cheese on top.

- Cover and simmer for 2-3 minutes or until the cheese is melted.

- Serve and enjoy.

You can also add some vegetables like mushrooms, peppers, or zucchini to increase the nutritional value of the dish.

Macros per serving

Calories: 600   Protein: 30g   Carbohydrates: 75g   Fat: 20g

Whole Wheat Pasta Primavera – 30 minutes

Ingredients:

- 8 oz whole wheat pasta

- 1 tbsp olive oil

- 1 red bell pepper, sliced

- 1 yellow bell pepper, sliced

- 1 onion, sliced

- 2 cloves of garlic, minced

- 1/2 cup frozen peas

- 1/4 cup grated Parmesan cheese

- Salt and pepper, to taste

- 2 tbsp of fresh parsley or basil, chopped into tiny pieces

Procedure:

Cook pasta. Drain and set aside.

In a pan, heat olive oil.

Add bell peppers, onion, and garlic to the skillet, and cook until softened, about 5 minutes.

Add the frozen peas and cook for another 2-3 minutes.

Toss in the cooked pasta and stir to combine.

Turn off the heat and stir in the Parmesan cheese, salt, and pepper.

Sprinkle with chopped parsley or basil and serve.

You can also add some protein like chicken, shrimp, or tofu to make it more complete meal.

Macros per serving

Calories: 400   Protein: 12g   Carbohydrates: 60g   Fat: 15g

Whole Wheat Pasta with Sausage and Peppers (2 servings) – 30 minutes

Ingredients:

- 8 oz whole wheat pasta
- 1 tbsp olive oil
- 1/2 lb sausage, sliced
- 1 red bell pepper, sliced
- 1 yellow bell pepper, sliced
- 1/4 tsp red pepper flakes
- 1/4 cup grated Parmesan cheese
- Salt and pepper to taste

Procedure:

- Cook the pasta. Drain and set aside.
- In a large pan, heat the olive oil. Put the sausages into the already heated pan and cook for 5 minutes.
- Add the bell peppers and red pepper flakes to the skillet and cook for another 5 minutes, or until the vegetables are softened.
- Add the cooked pasta an mix it all. Add salt and pepper to taste.
- Serve the pasta in bowls and sprinkle with grated Parmesan cheese.

Macros per serving

Calories: 550   Protein: 30g   Carbohydrates: 50g   Fat: 25g

—— ⸙ ——

LOW CARB DAY DINNER:

Grilled Chicken with Cauliflower Rice (2 servings) – 30 minutes

Ingredients:

- 2 boneless, skinless chicken breasts
- Salt and pepper, to taste
- 1 tbsp olive oil
- 1 head of cauliflower, grated
- 1 tbsp butter
- 1/4 cup grated Parmesan cheese
- 2 cloves of garlic, minced
- 2 tbsp chopped parsley

Procedure:

- Preheat grill to medium-high heat.
- Season chicken with salt and pepper.
- Grill chicken for about 6-8 minutes per side or until cooked through.
- Warm up a large pan and add olive oil.
- Put the garlic inside the heated pan and fry for 2 minutes.
- Add the grated cauliflower, butter, salt, and pepper to the skillet, and cook for about 5 minutes or until the cauliflower is tender.

- Stir in the Parmesan cheese and parsley.

- Serve the chicken with cauliflower rice on the side.

You can also add some vegetables like broccoli, bell peppers or mushrooms to add more variety and vitamins.

Macros per serving

Calories: 300   Protein: 35g   Carbohydrates: 5g   Fat: 20g

Baked Salmon with Green Beans (2 servings) – 30 minutes

Ingredients:

- 2 (6 oz) salmon fillets

- Salt and pepper, to taste

- 1 tbsp olive oil

- 1 lb green beans, trimmed

- 2 cloves of garlic, minced

- 2 tbsp lemon juice

- 1 tbsp chopped parsley

Procedure:

- Preheat the oven to 400F.

- Add salt and pepper to the salmon fillets.

- Place the salmon fillets in a baking dish and drizzle with olive oil.

- Bake for about 10-12 minutes, or until cooked through.

- In pan, warm up some olive oil.

- Put the garlic inside the heated pan and fry for 2 minutes.

- Add the green beans and cook for about 5 minutes or until tender-crisp.

- Add the lemon juice, salt, and pepper.

- Serve the salmon with green beans on the side and sprinkle with parsley.

You can also add some spices or herbs like thyme, dill or paprika to give the dish a different flavour.

Macros per serving

Calories: 300   Protein: 35g   Carbohydrates: 5g   Fat: 20g

Zucchini Noodles with Meat Sauce (2 servings) – 30 minutes

Ingredients:

- 2 medium zucchinis

- 1 tbsp olive oil

- 1 lb ground beef or turkey

- 1 onion, diced

- 2 cloves of garlic, minced

- 1 cup of your favourite marinara sauce

- Salt and pepper, to taste

- 2 tbsp grated Parmesan cheese

Procedure:

- Cut the zucchinis into noodles using a spiralizer or a julienne peeler.

- Warm up olive oil in a big pan.

- Add the ground meat, onion, and garlic and cook until browned, about 5-7 minutes.

- Add the marinara sauce and cook over low flame. Add salt and pepper to taste.

- Add the zucchini noodles to the skillet and cook until tender, about 2-3 minutes.

- Turn off the flame and add the Parmesan.

- Serve the zucchini noodles with meat sauce and top with grated Parmesan cheese.

You can also add some vegetables like mushrooms, bell peppers or spinach to add more variety and vitamins.

Macros per serving

Calories: 300   Protein: 20g   Carbohydrates: 10g   Fat: 20g

Spinach Stuffed Chicken Breasts (2 servings) – 30 minutes

Ingredients:

- 2 boneless, skinless chicken breasts

- Salt and pepper, to taste

- 2 cloves of garlic, minced

- 1/4 cup diced onion

- 4 cups fresh spinach leaves

- 1/4 cup crumbled feta cheese

- 2 tbsp olive oil

Procedure:

- Preheat the oven to 375F.

- Season chicken with salt and pepper.

- Warm up some olive oil in a large pan.

- Add the garlic and onion and cook for about 2-3 minutes or until softened.

- Add the spinach leaves and cook until wilted, about 2-3 minutes.

- Stir in the feta cheese and cook for another minute.

- Remove skillet from heat and let cool for a few minutes.

- Make a horizontal cut in the centre of each chicken breast to create a pocket.

- Stuff each chicken breast with the spinach mixture, secure with toothpicks if necessary.

- Place the chicken breasts in a baking dish.

- Bake for about 25-30 minutes or until cooked through.

You can also add some herbs or spices like thyme, oregano, or basil to give the dish a different flavour.

Macros per serving

Calories: 250   Protein: 25g   Carbohydrates: 5g   Fat: 15g

Baked Tilapia with Tomato and Caper Relish (2 servings) – 30 minutes

Ingredients:

- 2 tilapia fillets
- Salt and pepper, to taste
- 1 tbsp olive oil
- 1 cup cherry tomatoes, halved
- 1 tbsp capers
- 1 tbsp chopped parsley
- 1 tbsp lemon juice

Procedure:

- Preheat the oven to 375F.
- Add salt and pepper to taste to the tilapia fillets.
- Warm up some olive oil in a large pan.
- Add the cherry tomatoes and cook for 2-3 minutes or until they start to burst.
- Stir in capers, parsley, and lemon juice.
- Remove skillet from heat and let cool for a few minutes.
- Place the tilapia fillets in a baking dish.
- Spoon the tomato and caper relish over the fish.

- Bake for about 12-15 minutes or until fish is cooked through.

You can also add some herbs or spices like basil, oregano, or dill to give the dish a different flavour.

Macros per serving

Calories: 200   Protein: 25g   Carbohydrates: 4g   Fat: 10g

Pan-Seared Scallops with Spinach and Garlic (2 servings) – 25 minutes

Ingredients:

- 4 large scallops
- Salt and pepper, to taste
- 1 tbsp olive oil
- 1 tbsp butter
- 2 cloves of garlic, minced
- 2 cups fresh spinach leaves
- 1 tbsp lemon juice

Procedure:

- Season scallops with salt and pepper.
- Warm up some olive oil in a large pan.
- Add the scallops and cook for 2-3 minutes per side or until golden brown.
- Remove the scallops from the skillet and set aside.

- In the same skillet, add the butter and garlic and cook for 1-2 minutes or until fragrant.

- Add the spinach leaves and cook until wilted, about 2-3 minutes.

- Stir in the lemon juice.

- Return the scallops to the skillet and spoon the spinach and garlic mixture over the scallops.

- Cook for another minute or until heated through.

You can also add some herbs or spices like thyme, oregano, or basil to give the dish a different flavour.

Macros per serving

Calories: 200   Protein: 20g   Carbohydrates: 4g   Fat: 14g

Grilled Chicken with Cauliflower Mash and Green Beans (2 servings) – 30 minutes

Ingredients:

- 4 boneless, skinless chicken breasts

- Salt and pepper

- 1 head of cauliflower, chopped

- 1/4 cup heavy cream

- 2 cloves of garlic, minced

- 1/4 cup grated Parmesan cheese

- 1 lb green beans, trimmed

- 1 tbsp olive oil

- 1 lemon, juiced

Procedure:

- Warm up your grill or grill pan to medium heat. Incorporate salt and peppercorn to the poultry cutlets. Barbecue the fowl for a period ranging from 6 to 8 minutes on each side, or until it is fully cooked.

- While the chicken is grilling, bring a pot of water to a boil. Add the cauliflower and boil for 8-10 minutes, or until very tender. Drain and add the cauliflower to the pot with the chicken.

- Mash the cauliflower with a potato masher or an immersion blender. Stir in the heavy cream, garlic, and Parmesan cheese. Add salt and pepper to taste.

- In a separate pan, heat the olive oil over medium heat. Add the green beans and cook for 5-7 minutes, or until tender. Add salt, pepper, and lemon juice.

- Serve the chicken with the cauliflower mash and green beans on the side. Enjoy!

Macros per serving

Calories: 300   Protein: 42g   Carbohydrates: 10g   Fat: 12g

3.4. SNACKS

HIGH CARB DAY SNACKS:

Sweet Potato Fries (2 servings) – 30 minutes

Ingredients:

- 2 medium sweet potatoes
- 2 tbsp olive oil
- Salt and pepper, to taste
- 1 tsp paprika

Procedure:

- Preheat oven to 425F.
- Peel the sweet potatoes and give them the form of fries.
- Place the fries in a bowl and toss with olive oil, salt, pepper, and paprika.
- Put them in the oven.
- Bake for about 20-25 minutes or until crispy, flipping them halfway through.

You can also add some herbs or spices like cumin, oregano, or thyme to give the dish a different flavour.

Macros per serving

Calories: 200   Protein: 2g   Carbohydrates: 30g   Fat: 10g

Banana Chocolate Chip Muffins (6 servings) – 30 minutes

Ingredients:

- 1 cup all-purpose flour
- 1/2 cup whole wheat flour
- 1 tsp baking powder
- 1/4 tsp baking soda
- 1/2 tsp salt
- 1/2 cup granulated sugar
- 1/2 cup mashed ripe bananas (about 1 large banana)
- 1/4 cup vegetable oil
- 1 egg
- 1/4 cup milk
- 1 tsp vanilla extract
- 1/2 cup chocolate chips

Procedure:

- Preheat oven to 350F. Line a muffin tin with paper cups or grease it with cooking spray.
- In a medium bowl, mix together all the flours, baking soda, powder, and salt.
- In a separate large bowl, beat together sugar, banana, oil, egg, milk, and vanilla extract.
- Gradually incorporate the all the ingredients together, amalgamating them.
- Fold in the chocolate chips.

- Divide the batter evenly in the muffin cups that you already prepared.

- Bake for 20-25 minutes.

- Let cool on a wire rack for 5 minutes before removing the muffins from the tin.

You can also add some nuts or dried fruits to give the muffins a different flavour and texture.

Macros per serving

Calories: 200   Protein: 3g   Carbohydrates: 30g   Fat: 9g

Cheddar and Chive Biscuits (8 servings) – 30 minutes

Ingredients:

- 2 cups all-purpose flour
- 1 tablespoon baking powder
- 1/2 teaspoon salt
- 1/4 teaspoon black pepper
- 1/4 cup cold butter, divided into small pieces
- 1 cup cheddar cheese, grated
- 2 tablespoons chives, chopped
- 3/4 cup milk

Procedure:

- Preheat the oven to 425F.

- In a large bowl, mix together the flour, baking powder, and add salt and pepper.

- Using a pastry cutter or your fingers, cut in the butter until the mixture resembles coarse crumbs.

- Stir in the cheese and chives.

- Gradually pour in the milk, stirring until the dough comes together.

- Eject the dough onto a surface lightly dusted with flour and manipulate it through a process of compressing and stretching a limited number of times.

- Pat the dough out to a thickness of about 1/2 inch.

- Cut the dough into 2-inch circles or squares using a biscuit cutter or a knife.

- Arrange the small baked goods known as biscuits on the sheet for baking that has been previously readied.

- Bake for 12-15 minutes or until golden brown.

You can also add some bacon or jalapenos to give the biscuits a different flavour.

Macros per serving

Calories: 150   Protein: 5g   Carbohydrates: 15g   Fat: 8g

Blueberry and Cream Cheese Stuffed French Toast (2 servings) – 25 minutes

Ingredients:

- 4 slices of whole wheat bread
- 1/4 cup cream cheese
- 1/4 cup blueberries
- 2 eggs
- 1/4 cup milk
- 1 tsp vanilla extract
- 1 tbsp butter
- Maple syrup, for serving

Procedure:

- Preheat a griddle or a large skillet over medium heat.
- Spread cream cheese on two slices of bread and top each with blueberries.
- Place the remaining two slices of bread on top of the blueberries to make sandwiches.
- In a shallow dish, whisk together the eggs, milk, and vanilla extract.
- Dip the sandwiches into the egg mixture, making sure both sides are coated.
- Place the butter in the skillet and add the sandwiches. Cook each for 3 minutes.
- Serve hot with maple syrup on top.

You can also add some cinnamon or nutmeg to give the dish a different flavour.

Macros per serving

Calories: 400   Protein: 14g   Carbohydrates: 50g   Fat: 18g

Fruit and Yogurt Parfait (2 servings) – 15 minutes

Ingredients:

- 1 cup Greek yogurt
- 1/4 cup granola
- 1/2 cup mixed berries (strawberries, blueberries, raspberries)
- 1 tbsp honey

Procedure:

- In a small bowl, mix together the yogurt, granola, berries, and honey.
- Layer the mixture in 2 glasses, starting with yogurt, then granola, and then berries.
- Repeat the layers until all ingredients are used up.
- Serve immediately or put in the fridge and enjoy later.

You can also add some nuts or chocolate chips to give the parfait a different flavour.

Macros per serving

Calories: 250   Protein: 15g   Carbohydrates: 30g   Fat: 5g

Cheesy Garlic Bread (2 servings) – 25 minutes

Ingredients:

- 2 slices of whole wheat bread
- 2 tbsp butter, room temperature
- 2 cloves of garlic, minced
- 1/4 cup grated mozzarella cheese
- 1 tbsp grated Parmesan cheese
- 1 tbsp chopped parsley

Procedure:

- Preheat the oven to 350F.
- Mix together butter, garlic, mozzarella, Parmesan and parsley in a small bowl.
- Use a knife to put the butter mixture on the slices of bread.
- Place the slices of bread on the baking sheet and bake for 8-10 minutes or until the cheese is melted and the bread is golden brown.
- Serve warm.

You can also add some herbs or spices to give the bread a different flavour.

Macros per serving

Calories: 250   Protein: 10g   Carbohydrates: 30g   Fat: 12g

LOW CARB DAY SNACKS

Devilled Eggs (2 servings) – 25 minutes

Ingredients:

- 4 eggs
- 2 tbsp mayonnaise
- 1 tsp Dijon mustard
- 1/4 tsp paprika
- Salt and pepper to taste

Procedure:

- Put the eggs in a saucepan and cover with water and boil.
- Simmer for 8-10 minutes, then transfer the eggs to a bowl of ice water to cool.
- Remove the eggshells and cut them in half.
- Remove the yolks and mash them in a small bowl with mayonnaise, mustard, paprika, salt and pepper.
- transfer the yolk amalgamation back into the egg albumen.
- Garnish with paprika or chopped chives and serve.

You can also add some herbs or spices to give the devilled eggs a different flavour.

Macros per serving

Calories: 150   Protein: 8g   Carbohydrates: 1g   Fat: 13g

Celery and Peanut Butter Snack (2 servings) – 10 minutes

Ingredients:

- 4 celery stalks

- 2 tbsp natural peanut butter

- 1 tbsp chopped peanuts

Procedure:

- Wash and dry the celery stalks.

- Put some peanut butter on the celery.

- Top with chopped peanuts.

- Serve and enjoy.

Macros per serving

Calories: 150   Protein: 5g   Carbohydrates: 5g   Fat: 12g

Spicy Jalapeno Cheddar Bites (2 servings) – 25 minutes

Ingredients:

- 1/2 cup almond flour

- 1/2 cup grated cheddar cheese

- 1/4 cup diced jalapeno

- 1 egg

- Salt and pepper to taste

Procedure:

- Preheat the oven to 350F.

- In a mixing bowl, combine almond flour, cheddar cheese, diced jalapeno, egg, salt and pepper. Mix until well combined.

- Roll the mixture into small balls and place them on the baking sheet.

- Bake for 10-15 minutes.

- Serve warm.

These bites are low in carbohydrates, high in protein and packed with flavour. You can also add some herbs or spices to give the bites a different flavour.

Macros per serving

Calories: 150   Protein: 8g   Carbohydrates: 3g   Fat: 12g

―――――――⟨ ⁓ ⟩―――――――

Cucumber and Cream Cheese Bites (2 servings) – 15 minutes

Ingredients:

- 1 cucumber

- 1/4 cup cream cheese

- 2 tbsp chopped chives
- Salt and pepper to taste

Procedure:

- Slice the cucumber into 1/4-inch rounds.
- Mix cream cheese, chives, salt, and pepper in a small bowl.
- Spread the mixture on top of the cucumber slices.
- Serve and enjoy.

This snack is easy to prepare, low in calories and carbohydrates, and high in healthy fats. You can also add some herbs or spices to give the bites a different flavour.

Macros per serving

Calories: 90   Protein: 2g   Carbohydrates: 2g   Fat: 8g

Spicy Parmesan Zucchini Fries (2 servings) – 25 minutes

Ingredients:

- 2 medium zucchinis
- 1/4 cup grated Parmesan cheese
- 1 tsp paprika
- 1 tsp garlic powder
- Salt and pepper to taste

- 2 tbsp olive oil

Procedure:

- Preheat the oven to 425F.

- Cut the zucchinis into fry-shaped pieces.

- In a small mixing bowl, combine Parmesan cheese, paprika, garlic powder, salt and pepper.

- Place the zucchini fries on the baking sheet and drizzle with olive oil.

- Sprinkle the Parmesan cheese mixture over the fries, ensuring they are evenly coated.

- Bake for 15-20 minutes.

- Serve and enjoy.

These zucchini frites are a palatable and nutritious low-carbohydrate titbit that can be relished at any juncture of the diurnal cycle.

Macros per serving

Calories: 150   Protein: 4g   Carbohydrates: 4g   Fat: 13g

Crispy Baked Parmesan and Herb Chicken Tenders (2 servings) – 25 minutes

Ingredients:

- 4 boneless, skinless chicken tenders

- 1/4 cup grated Parmesan cheese

- 1 tsp dried basil

- 1 tsp dried oregano

- Salt and pepper to taste

- 1 egg

- 1/4 cup almond flour

Procedure:

- Preheat the oven to 425F.

- In a small mixing bowl, combine Parmesan cheese, basil, oregano, salt, and pepper.

- In another plate, beat the egg.

- Dip each chicken tender in the beaten egg, then coat in the almond flour mixture.

- Place the chicken tenders on the baking sheet and sprinkle with the Parmesan cheese mixture, ensuring they are evenly coated.

- Bake for 15-20 minutes.

- Serve and enjoy.

These chicken tenders are a delicious low-carb snack that can be enjoyed at any time of the day. You can adjust the seasoning to your preference and serve with your favourite dipping sauce.

Macros per serving

Calories: 250   Protein: 25g   Carbohydrates: 3g   Fat: 16g

3.5. Easy food prep if you don't have time

Carb Cycling can be a highly effective method for attaining fitness objectives, however, its demands for meal preparation during the week can prove to be a substantial time burden. For those who have limited time, there are a few easy food preparation techniques that can help make carb cycling more manageable.

Meal prepping: One of the most important steps in food preparation is meal planning. This means deciding in advance what meals you will be eating for the week, and making a grocery list accordingly. This can help you save time and money and ensure that you always have the ingredients you need on hand. One of the most efficacious means of conserving time during the week is to perform your sustenance preparation on the weekends. This may encompass the culinary preparation and apportioning of your comestibles for the week, so that all that is necessary is to retrieve and depart during the week. Here are some guidelines for achieving that.

1. Batch cooking: Batch cooking is another useful strategy for food preparation. This means cooking a large batch of food, such as a big pot of chili or a tray of baked chicken. It can serve as an efficacious means of ensuring availability of a multitude of sustenance in a prompt manner. This can be especially helpful for high-carb days when you need to eat more food and can save time and make it easy to have healthy meals on hand during the week.

2. Crockpot cooking: Crockpots are a great way to cook a variety of meals with minimal preparation. You can set it in the morning, and by dinner time, you will have a hot meal ready to eat.

3. Freezing meals: Advance culinary preparation and refrigerant preservation can be a viable stratagem for augmenting one's weekly temporal efficiency. This may encompass the congelation of discretely portioned dishes such as hotpots,

broths, and ragouts, facilitating rapid thawing and subsequent re-heating. Always remember to Store food properly: Use airtight containers to store your food in the fridge or freezer. This will help keep the food fresh and prevent spoilage.

4. Use of leftovers: Take advantage of leftovers from previous meals, it can be a fast and easy way to have a meal ready to go. Cook extra portions of your meals so that you have leftovers to take with you to work or school the next day. This will mitigate the expenditures of both time and funds while also assisting in adhering to the regimen of alternating carbohydrate intake.

5. Plan ahead: Before you start cooking, make a plan of what meals you want to prepare for the week. This will help you to make a grocery list, make sure you have all the ingredients you need and save time on the weekend. Prepping in advance also means doing things like washing and cutting vegetables, cooking grains, and prepping proteins ahead of time. This can help to obviate the need for expended time allocation throughout the week and enhance your adherence to the regimen of carb-cycling.

6. Make a grocery list. Formulate a list of required ingredients by compiling a grocery list after you have established your meal plan. This will aid in maintaining order and deter impulsive purchases.

7. Employ the utilization of ingredients that can be utilized in numerous culinary preparations: For example, if you are cooking ground beef, cook enough for multiple meals, like tacos and spaghetti.

8. Employ the utilization of a pressure cooker: Pressure cookers can cut cooking time significantly, great for cooking grains, beans and meats. These appliances make it easy to prepare large quantities of food with minimal effort. You can throw

your ingredients in the morning, and come home to a hot and ready meal.

9. Use a sheet pan: Sheet pans are perfect for baking multiple items at once, like chicken, fish, and vegetables.

10. Engage in substantial culinary production: Make large batches of food and portion them out for the week, like a big pot of chili or a tray of baked chicken.

11. Invest in a good food processor: A food processor will save you a lot of time on chopping and dicing vegetables.

12. Use a slow cooker: Slow cookers are perfect for preparing meals in advance, you can put all ingredients in the morning and by the evening you will have a hot meal ready to serve.

13. Formulate pre-prepared meals, ahead of time: Another strategy for food preparation is to make meals in advance that can be easily reheated later. This can include things like casseroles, soups, and stews, which can be made in bulk and then portioned out for later use. This can be especially helpful for low-carb days, when you may not have as much time to cook. Assemble meals that can be stored in the refrigerator or freezer, like casseroles or sandwiches, so they are easy to grab and go during the week.

14. Use frozen vegetables: Frozen vegetables are a great time-saver. Frozen fruits and vegetables possess a similar nutritional value as their fresh counterparts and are frequently more commodious. They are already trimmed and purged, rendering them convenient to incorporate into your nourishment, and can be utilized in multiple culinary preparations. And if you prefer fresh vegetables chop and prepare them in advance, so they are ready to use when you need them.

15. Marinate your protein: Marinating your protein in advance allows the flavours to penetrate, making the meal more flavourful and delicious.

16. Cook grains in bulk: Cook grains like rice, quinoa, and oats in bulk on the weekend, then store them in the fridge or freezer for easy use during the week.

17. Make your own salad dressings: Making your own salad dressings can be healthier and more cost-effective.

18. Prep your protein: Prepare a substantial quantity of protein sources such as poultry, seafood, or bean curd and preserve it within the refrigeration apparatus or cryogenic storage for expeditious utilization throughout the week.

19. Make your own snacks: Instead of buying pre-made snacks, make your own, like granola bars, trail mix, or roasted nuts.

20. Use leftovers: Use leftovers from dinner to make lunch for the next day, for example, use leftover grilled chicken to make a salad.

21. Meal plan: Make a meal plan for the week and stick to it, so you know what meals you need to prepare, and you can make sure you have all ingredients on hand.

22. Mix and match: Have some basic ingredients on hand that can be mixed and matched to create different meals throughout the week.

23. Get creative: Meal prep doesn't have to be boring, get creative with your recipes and ingredients to keep things interesting.

24. Be flexible: Remember that things don't always go as planned, so be flexible and have backup options in case something falls through.

By incorporating these techniques into your carb cycling routine, you can save time during the week and make the process more manageable.

In conclusion effective food preparation is crucial for success with carb cycling. By planning meals in advance, prepping ingredients, making make-ahead meals, batch cooking, and using leftovers, you can save time and ensure that you always have healthy, nutrient-dense meals on hand. Additionally, tips for busy individuals such as freezing meals and using slow cookers and pressure cookers can help make the process more manageable.

PART FOUR

F.A.Q.

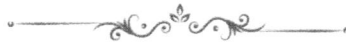

1. Can I do carb cycling while pregnant or breastfeeding. It is imperative to seek medical counsel before embarking upon any new dietetic regimen or physical fitness program during pregnancy or lactation. The methodology of carb cycling may not be suitable for all individuals during these phases, hence, it is crucial to communicate with one's healthcare professional regarding one's unique necessities.

2. Can I do carb cycling while following a vegetarian or vegan diet? Yes, you can adapt carb cycling to fit a vegetarian or vegan diet. Instead of relying on meat as a primary source of protein, you can incorporate plant-based proteins such as beans, lentils, and tofu.

3. I am not losing weight while carb cycling. Why? There could be several reasons for this. It is imperative to guarantee that the correct proportion of macronutrients is adhered to, commensurate with one's objectives and level of physical activity. Additionally, make sure you are accurately tracking your food intake and not overeating. It may be prudent to engage the services of a competent dietary expert, such as a registered dietitian, to assess and modify your dietary regimen as deemed necessary.

4. I am feeling sluggish and tired on low carb days. What can I do? It is common to feel low on energy on low carb days,

especially if you are not used to eating a low carb diet. To address this issue, it is imperative to ingest adequate amounts of protein and wholesome lipids during low-carbohydrate days to preserve satiety and contentment. Additionally, incorporating more nutrient-dense foods such as leafy greens, nuts, and seeds can help provide energy.

5. Can I do carb cycling while training for a marathon? Carb cycling can be challenging for athletes who need a consistent intake of carbohydrates to fuel their intense training. It is important to consult with a sports dietitian to ensure that your diet is meeting your energy needs during intense training.

6. Can I do carb cycling while following a low-FODMAP diet? The adaptation of Carb Cycling to a low-FODMAP regimen may pose difficulties in attaining the required intake of carbohydrates. It is advisable to seek the counsel of a professional nutritionist to guarantee that adequate amounts of carbohydrates are being consumed whilst adhering to a low-FODMAP diet.

7. I'm having trouble sticking to the plan. What can I do? Carb cycling can be challenging to stick to, especially in the beginning. Make sure to plan your meals and snacks in advance and have healthy options readily available. It may also be helpful to track your progress and see how far you have come. Remember, it is okay to slip up, the important thing is to get back on track as soon as possible.

CONCLUSION

In summation, the technique of carb cycling involves oscillating between periods of ample and limited carbohydrate ingestion. This method of eating can help to boost weight loss, improve athletic performance, and increase muscle mass and is based on the principle that by manipulating carbohydrate intake, you can optimize hormone levels, improve insulin sensitivity, and improve overall health. Nevertheless, it is crucial to bear in mind that carb cycling may not be a fitting approach for all individuals, and it is advisable to seek the guidance of a medical professional prior to implementing substantial modifications to one's nutritional regimen. The preparation of meals in advance is an efficacious method for rendering the implementation of carb cycling more feasible, particularly for those with hectic lifestyles. By taking the time to prepare meals in advance, you can ensure that you have healthy and nutritious options available throughout the week, without having to spend hours in the kitchen. With proper methodology, alternation of carbohydrate intake through carb cycling can prove to be a viable means of accomplishing health and fitness objectives.

In this book, we covered the basics of carb cycling, including what it is, how it works, and the benefits it can offer. We also discussed how to calculate your daily carbohydrate needs, how to plan your meals and snacks, and how to track your progress. Additionally, we proffered a plethora of culinary formulae, physical exertion regimens, and alternative recommendations to aid you in integrating the regimen of carb cycling into your modus vivendi.

It must be remembered that carb cycling is a versatile technique, and can be adjusted to suit one's specific requirements and inclinations.

It is also imperative to acknowledge that carb cycling is not an approach that accommodates every person, and may not be apt for those with specific health issues, pregnant or lactating women, or those with a low body weight.

A salient benefit of carb cycling is the possibility of systematic carbohydrate consumption, thereby mitigating feelings of deprivation and enhancing compliance with the regimen. Furthermore, by alternating between days with high and low carbohydrate intake, it can help to thwart the body from becoming acclimated to a low carbohydrate diet and reduce the rate of metabolism.

When it comes to meal prepping for carb cycling, it's important to plan ahead and have a variety of healthy options available. This encompasses the provision of nourishment that is rich in proteins and wholesome lipids, as well as having a plethora of low-carbohydrates and high-carbohydrates alternatives obtainable. Meal prepping can also help to save time and money, as well as reducing the likelihood of making unhealthy food choices.

In synthesis, the technique of carb cycling represents a dietary methodology that can yield positive outcomes for those who aspire to augment their physical appearance and athletic prowess. Nevertheless, prior to effecting any substantial modification to one's regimen, it is imperative to seek advice from a healthcare practitioner. With the right approach and meal prepping, carb cycling can be a convenient and effective way to achieve your health and fitness goals.

In summation, carb cycling is a widespread and efficacious method for controlling body weight and augmenting overall well-being. By oscillating between days of abundant and meagre carbohydrate intake, one can still partake of carbohydrates while concurrently stimulating fat reduction and muscle accretion. Nonetheless, it is imperative to heed the fact that carb cycling should be adjusted to your personal requirements and aspirations, and should be performed under the supervision of a medical expert. Furthermore, it is not a miracle solution and requires a lot of effort and discipline.

When it comes to meal preparation, it can be difficult to find the time to cook during the week. However, by spending a couple of hours on the weekend to prepare and portion out meals, you can make your life much easier during the week. Some tips include:

- Preparing a big batch of protein, such as chicken or fish

- Cooking a variety of vegetables to have on hand

- Prepping healthy snacks, such as cut-up fruits or veggies

- Using a slow cooker or pressure cooker to make meals in advance

- Investing in good quality containers to store the food.

By following these tips and incorporating carb cycling into your diet, you can take control of your nutrition and achieve your goals in a sustainable way. Everyone's needs and goals are different, so it's important to adjust your plan as needed. If you find that you are not seeing the results you want or are experiencing negative side effects, it may be necessary to make adjustments to your plan.

In order to persevere along your itinerary of alternating carbohydrate intake, it is crucial to sustain inspiration and responsibility. One means of achieving this objective is through the establishment of both near-term and distant aspirations. By setting specific, measurable, and achievable goals, you can stay focused and motivated. Additionally, it can be helpful to find a support group, whether it's friends, family, or an online community, to share your experiences and get tips and advice.

To summarize, the utilization of a cyclical variation in carbohydrate intake constitutes a potent dietary strategy that can assist in attaining your objectives relating to weight reduction, muscular augmentation, and athletic proficiency. By understanding the principles of carb cycling, planning your meals and snacks, and tracking your progress, you can optimize your hormone levels, improve insulin sensitivity, and improve your overall health. With dedication, consistency, and patience, you can continue your carb cycling journey and achieve the results you desire.

.

Made in the USA
Las Vegas, NV
28 August 2023